Surviving and Thriving with Colon Cancer

A Comprehensive Guide providing Home Remedies for Promoting Digestive Health and Preventing Colon Issues

Ted Whitworth

D1127922

GET YOUR FREE E-BOOK!

Do you want to escape the unending cycle of pharmaceutical drugs and feel truly healthy? Then give nature a chance. Find out how beautiful-looking herbs can cure and prevent diseases and how to use herbs effectively by signing up for your free copy today!

VISIT: www.tedmedicinal.com

Table of Contents

Introduction

At some point or another, we have all suffered from digestive problems. And whether they are chronic or only occur once in a while, they are uncomfortable and sometimes even debilitating. So certainly, it is necessary in some cases to resort to a colon cleansing to help us make the situation lighter.

You may be plagued with everything when the colon does not work properly, from headaches, low energy, and fatigue to swelling, gas, and constipation. This is because this part of our digestive system does the important job of processing nutrients from foodstuffs and removing solid waste from the body.

The colon, or large intestine, is a tube that measures about 5 feet in length and is responsible for expelling waste from the body. Lifestyle factors, particularly the nutrition in what we eat, directly affect the inner mucous lining of the colon and the outer muscle wall. As a result, the large intestine receives food processed in the esophagus, stomach, and small intestine. By this time, the body has taken in most of the nutrients it needs, and fermentation helps it take in the rest. Following completion of this process, the colon expels the waste.

Consuming high-fiber foods is beneficial because it helps the colon's lining work more efficiently, resulting in more rapid and painless removal. Unfortunately, many modern diets consist primarily of processed foods with low fiber content, which hinder the colon's ability to function normally. Because waste typically leaves layers of residue and debris behind, which react differently with intestinal mucous based on their content, this is one of the major root causes in almost all cases of poor colon health. In addition, insufficient fiber in the diet can weaken the muscle walls of the colon and restrict bowel movement by creating a thick coating that is difficult to expel. The fiber in food can help clear the colon of this waste, allowing the organ to function more optimally.

We have all heard the adage, "You are what you eat," and while this may not always be true, it certainly rings true here. The demands of modern life leave us with little time to devote to meal preparation, making it difficult to meet the nutritional requirements outlined by our evolutionary ancestors. Instead, we rely on technological advances in the food processing industry to save time and effort. Additionally, while digestive difficulties like overindulging in alcohol or not eating enough fiber may increase enjoyment at the moment, they make digestion and elimination more laborious in the long run. Over time, the colon can become overwhelmed by the accumulation of these toxins from waste.

This book is what you have been looking for. Let's get started!

Chapter 1: Understanding Colon?

Although the colon is often referred to as the "large intestine" or "large bowel," it is only a small portion of the larger intestine. However, the large intestine is likely among the most crucial organs in the digestive system. The digestive tract, also known as the gastrointestinal system, is the network of organs that aids in the breakdown and absorption of solid and liquid foods. (This entails eating, swallowing, digesting, and passing the food through one's system.)

The cecum, colon, rectum, and anus are the four sections that together form the large intestine. Colon length alone can add half a meter to an adult's total length.

When the cecum connects to the ileum at the very end of the small intestine in the lower right of the abdomen, this marks the beginning of the colon. When the colon reaches its final six inches, the tissues it contains move into the rectal region, which is commonly known as the rectum.

The colon is a large, hollow tube with the appearance of an inverted 'U.' It consists of these four sections: An example of an ascending colon is the beginning of a colon. Moving upward from the right side of the abdomen, this section begins in the cecum and continues to the right.

After traveling up and in for about 20 to 25 centimeters, the colon turns horizontal and stretches across the upper abdomen for another 30 to 60 centimeters, a position known as a transverse colon. The sigmoid colon is that portion of the colon that makes a sharp right curve immediately before the rectum.

Do you have good colon health?

Have a Self-check

Did you know a chart can tell if your stool shapes are okay?

It's called the Bristol stool chart. This chart has two types of standard stool shapes. One is shaped like a brown sausage with cracks, and the other is a smooth brown snake shape. If you have too many breaks and it's more difficult to pass than usual, that's constipation.

There are two degrees of constipation before it turns into a severe problem. The first degree is when the stool has more bumps and cracks, and the final degree is when there are separated, hard pieces of stool.

If your stool lacks shape, is loose, and comes with an uncomfortable feeling, that's diarrhea.

There are three degrees of constipation before it turns into a severe problem. The first degree is when the stool cannot hold itself together. The second degree is when the stool becomes mushy and contains more liquid than in regular bowel movements. The final degree is when the stool becomes a liquid consistency, and you experience painful bowel movements.

The Colors of Stool Can Also Differ

For good colon health, you want to be looking for brown, but if there is a little green, that is okay.

- When stools are mainly green, the food waste has passed through the colon too quickly, or your diet has introduced a lot of green vegetables in a short period.

- When stools are mainly yellow, the gastrointestinal system might have fat absorption problems.

- If your bowel movements are white, black, or red, go to the emergency room. You may be experiencing internal bleeding, and something serious may be happening in your gastrointestinal system.

How the Digestive System Works

Many of us are unaware of our digestive system because it works and heals itself automatically. The lining of our digestive tract can repair or change itself every 3 to 5 days. The only time we truly feel concerned about it is when we feel pain in our stomach. It is extremely important to take good care of our digestive system, regardless of whether we feel this pain or not, and the first step to a healthier tract is to understand how it works.

Imagine the digestive system as a hose that starts from your mouth and ends in your anus. It is approximately 25 to 35 feet long, and everything you put in your mouth goes through it. The process that enables the food to travel through your digestive tract is performed by an automated muscular contraction called "peristalsis." As the food travels through this tube, it goes through a series of processes to extract cells that your body will use for energy, healing, and sustenance. A blockage or any other irregularity in this process will cause pain in your stomach. It will also disable the digestive system from breaking down foods and transferring the essential nutrients to the rest of your body. You may have heard the modern-day saying, "Do not treat your mouth like a garbage can." This apparently means that you should watch what you eat, which holds so much truth. The brain is most responsible for the health of the digestive system because it is the one that makes the decisions as to the kinds of food to consume. Therefore, whenever you see and smell something, your brain will signal the different parts of your body to want this particular food and to consume it.

To give you a simple overview of how our digestive system works, the main parts and their functions will be discussed below:

The Mouth

The entryway to the digestive system is the mouth. It is where the food is placed, lubricated, and broken down by our tongue, teeth, and saliva. It is then pushed deeper into the esophagus.

The Esophagus

The esophagus is also referred to as the food pipe and is located just below the throat. It is where the food will continue to travel via peristalsis. Even if you are lying down or turned upside down, peristalsis is strong enough to continue pushing your food into your stomach.

The Stomach

Strong muscular contractions and the release of powerful acids and enzymes continue to break down the food inside the stomach. After going through the stomach, the food will look like boiled oatmeal. This will travel through a small ring of muscle called the "pylorus."

The Pylorus

This little muscle is important because it connects the stomach and the small intestine. It ensures that the small intestine does not become overwhelmed by the processed food from the stomach.

The Small Intestine

The food continues to be broken down in the small intestine, both physically by the muscular contractions and chemically by the enzymes secreted in this part of the digestive tract. Our body secretes different types of enzymes to digest different kinds of nutrients from food.

The small intestine can stretch to approximately 15 feet long and is covered with a lining named "villi." Upon closer inspection, the villi are covered with tiny, hairlike protrusions called "microvilli." These are responsible for transferring the nutrients from the food into your bloodstream.

The initial part of the small intestine is called the "duodenum," and it is this place where much of the enzymes excreted by the pancreas and bile from the liver are mixed in with the food for further digestion. In addition, certain nutrients, such as calcium, zinc, and iron, are immediately absorbed at this point.

The rest of the small intestine comprises the "jejunum," which makes up around 40 percent of it, and the "ileum," which is 60 percent. Some foods that are more difficult to digest are pushed into these parts for further absorption of nutrients.

The Large Intestine

You might already know that food is not completely processed in the small intestine because another part of the digestive system continues to do this job. It is the large intestine, or what others call our "colon." It measures about 5 feet.

There are many special types of bacteria within the large intestine, and they are very important in breaking down carbohydrates that the small intestine was unable to do. They also work on synthesizing some of the B vitamins and vitamin K. It is also important to know that this process produces gas.

When food reaches the end of the large intestine, it has already degraded into feces, which is mostly water and indigestible organic matter containing bacteria and dead villi cells. Next, it travels to the rectum, where it builds up until your bowels decide to push it out.

Now that you have a better understanding of how the digestive system works, it is also essential to know how the different nutrients in food are absorbed. Below are the main nutrients and how our digestive system breaks them down and absorbs them into the bloodstream. Understanding these processes is also important to help prepare you for developing and creating a diet for a healthier digestive system.

Protein

Meat, eggs, and beans contain a lot of protein. After consuming these foods, the body needs to digest them with enzymes before absorbing the protein used to develop and repair your body tissues. First, the stomach starts digesting the food with enzymes. After this, it proceeds to the small intestine and is further broken down into amino acids by pancreatic juice and muscular contractions. The amino acids are then absorbed into the bloodstream and distributed throughout the body.

Vitamins

Vitamins are mostly absorbed through our small intestine. There are two types of vitamins: water-soluble (the B vitamins and vitamin C) and fat-soluble (A, D, E, and K).

Water-soluble vitamins are not stored easily, and excessive amounts consumed are expelled from the body in the urine. On the other hand, fat-soluble vitamins are stored both in the liver and the fatty tissues.

Carbohydrates

You can get carbohydrates from bread, rice, pasta, potatoes, beans, fruits, and vegetables. They contain mostly starch, sugars, and fiber.

The digestive system breaks down starch with enzymes in the saliva and pancreatic juice. It turns it into maltose, which then splits into glucose molecules that the liver absorbs into the bloodstream to store energy.

Sugars are broken down by enzymes in the villi and turn sucrose into glucose, fructose, and sometimes lactose (from milk). These are also absorbed into the bloodstream.

Fiber continues to travel throughout the digestive tract as it cannot be digested. There are mainly two types of fiber: soluble (which easily breaks down in the water and turns into gelatin in the intestines) and insoluble (which does not change as it passes through the digestive tract).

Fats

A lot of your energy comes from fat molecules. Fat is broken down by your digestive system by dissolving it into watery matter via bile acids from your liver and pancreatic juice. The broken-down, smaller molecules are composed of cholesterol and fatty acids. These combine with bile acids and are transferred through the lymphatic system to the chest veins . After that, it is brought to storage depots in certain parts of your body.

Water and Salt

The water and salt inside us are taken from our food and drink and combined with the excretions of our digestive glands. As a result, much of the matter that is absorbed through our small intestine is water and dissolved salt.

What Functions Does the Colon Serve in the Body?

The colon is responsible for the digestive process's final stages. Its three primary functions in the body are as follows:

- Absorbing residual water and electrolytes from previously digested food. • Absorbing and storing food remains that were not digested in the small intestine, such as vitamin K. Processing indigestible materials such as fiber.

- Storing and later removing solid waste known as feces. Feces is an indigestible mixture of fiber, water, mucus, bacteria, and other substances.
- The colon performs the following tasks to perform these functions:
- The small intestine transports partially digested food to the colon. This food is in the form of a liquid.
- Bacteria in the colon break down this partially digested food into smaller constituents.
- The colon's epithelium, or inner lining, absorbs nutrients from the broken-down, smaller parts.
- After the nutrients have been absorbed, what is left is combined to form feces. Feces is still semi-solid.
- The epithelium produces mucus to help it pass easily through the rectum and anus.
- As feces enters the rectum, it is stored there until the rectum is full. At that point, the brain signals the body to begin pushing the feces out. Toxins are commonly found in feces, so it is critical to expel them from the body regularly.

Bacteria or bowel flora in the colon play an important role in this process. Their job is to feed on fiber, break it down, and absorb all nutrients. They also keep the pH balanced and prevent the growth of harmful bacteria.

Nearly 60 different types of bacteria live in the colon. The majority of these bacteria are beneficial, such as Bacillus coli and Acidophilus. However, the colon is home to a few pathogenic bacteria. Both exist in a healthy balance here, keeping an individual hale and hearty.

Diseases of the Colon

The disease of the colon can range from the presence of cancerous masses to the uncomfortable symptoms of Irritable Bowel Syndrome. In addition, poor digestion can necessitate surgery or cause a person to alter their diet and lifestyle radically.

Benign Growths

Benign masses in the colon include neoplasms or tumors that do not recur after removal. These growths contain clumps of tissue that serve no purpose and do not spread, but they compromise the surrounding tissue's health. As a result, they grow more slowly and are less likely to cause problems.

Any mass of this type can also be detected during a colonoscopy and will either be removed or biopsied during the procedure.

Diverticulitis

Diverticulitis is caused by eating a diet low in fiber. A diverticuli is a ruptured spot in the colon that causes an infection in adjacent tissue.

The subsequent pressure then leads to sacs that bulge or push outward from the colon. A single site is called a diverticulum, while multiple affected areas are diverticula.

These ruptures and bulges can occur anywhere in the colon but are typically located toward the sigmoid's end.

Symptoms of their presence include bleeding, constipation, abdominal cramping, and potentially colon obstruction. In addition, the abdomen may be tender and painful when infection sets in, and the individual may run a fever.

Other symptoms can include vomiting, bloating, abnormal urination (frequent and painful), and rectal bleeding.

Diverticulitis is most common in the world's developed nations and less prevalent in Africa and Asia. People younger than 40 rarely develop the condition, but 15% of people aged 60 or more in the United States suffer from the problem.

Recommended courses of treatment vary with the severity of any number of acute episodes. A liquid or low-fiber diet with antibiotics may be recommended if the episode is mild.

Individuals at high risk of infection or repeated episodes may face surgery to remove the diseased portion of the intestine. In addition, a temporary colostomy may be necessary in very severe cases until the intestine has properly healed.

Polyps

Polyps are the most common non-cancerous growths found on the colon's lining. They are small balls of abnormal cells attached to stalks. Typically, the masses are 2 mm to 5 cm or more in diameter.

It is important to determine the nature of the cells forming the polyp to judge the risk of cancer developing accurately. For example, metaplastic polyps do not present a danger, but adenomatous polyps can become malignant.

Even in a healthy colon, about 10% of the cells exhibit apparent abnormalities. In most cases, however, these cells die a "pre-programmed" death via apoptosis and fall harmlessly into the lumen or bowel cavity.

If a polyp grows to a diameter of 2 cm, bleeding from the anus will usually begin, with evidence visible in underwear, on toilet paper, or via black or red-streaked stools.

Either diarrhea or constipation may be present for more than a week at a time. Diarrhea will be profuse and watery, leading to muscle weakness due to potassium deficiency. Severe abdominal pain is possible. Polyps can be detected during a colonoscopy that examines the entire bowel length. The growths may be removed during that procedure while the patient is already sedated.

Other diagnostic procedures include a sigmoidoscopy (which examines the last third of the colon), a barium enema, and a digital examination.

Although dietary changes are not considered effective by many experts, the risk of polyps has been significantly lower in non-smokers, people who do not consume fatty foods and maintain a normal weight, individuals who exercise regularly, and those who do not drink.

Ulcerative Colitis

Ulcerative colitis is a form of inflammatory bowel disease characterized by open sores or ulcers that cause constant diarrhea mixed with blood. The condition is often confused with Crohn's Disease and Irritable Bowel Syndrome.

Ulcerative colitis is, however, an intermittent disease. Patients may go for extended periods during which they suffer no symptoms whatsoever.

The incidence rate is approximately one in every twenty people per 100,000 people annually, with a higher number of cases in the developed world (particularly in affluent nations.)

There is no known cause for ulcerative colitis, although a genetic susceptibility is strongly assumed. In addition, environmental factors can trigger an episode, but the condition is not believed to be caused by diet.

Diet modifications can, however, reduce the degree of discomfort experienced. Typical treatment involves anti-inflammatory medications.

Crohn's Disease

Crohn's Disease (Chrohn's Syndrome or Regional Enteritis) is also an inflammatory condition of the bowel but may affect any part of the gastrointestinal tract from the mouth to the anus.

The disease is responsible for a broad range of symptoms, including, but not limited to, abdominal pain, diarrhea (often bloody), vomiting (which may be continuous), and weight loss.

Crohn's is caused by the interaction of multiple environmental, immunological, and bacterial factors.

Genetic susceptibility is a chronic inflammatory disease in which the body's immune system begins to attack the GI tract.

There is no cure, and remissions are never certain. As a result, the best approach supported by conventional medicine is to combine medication with lifestyle and dietary changes.

Stress reduction and moderate exercise are also important components of management.

Surgery is not recommended; once controlled, Crohn's can be managed long-term with moderate success.

Celiac Disease

Celiac disease is an autoimmune disorder of the small intestine that affects people who are genetically predisposed to it It can occur at any time, from middle infancy to old age.

The most obvious symptoms are digestive pain and discomfort, marked by chronic constipation and diarrhea.

Children with Celiac disease will fail to thrive, and almost all patients will, at some point, exhibit anemia and extreme fatigue. In addition, vitamin deficiencies are common because the small intestine cannot properly absorb nutrients.

The condition is caused by an allergic reaction to the gluten protein, which must be completely removed from the diet for the patient to exhibit real recovery. Celiac is thought to affect about 1 in 1,750 people worldwide, but in the United States, it is seen in 1 out of 105.

Colorectal Cancer

More commonly called colon or bowel cancer, colorectal cancer occurs in the presence of an uncontrolled mass of cell growth in the colon, rectum, or appendix.

The most obvious signs are rectal bleeding and anemia, with marked changes in bowel habits and weight loss. The disease starts in the lining of the bowel but, if not detected, can spread through the muscle layers and then through the bowel wall.

Colonoscopy or sigmoidoscopy is recommended as a screening mechanism for ages 50-75. If the disease is confined within the colon wall, it is curable with surgery.

If cancer has spread, treatment focuses on life extension with chemotherapy and other measures to enhance the quality of life.

Colorectal cancer is the third most-diagnosed cancer in the world. Sixty percent of cases, however, are found in the developed world.

Gastrointestinal Defense Mechanisms

The human gastrointestinal system has many self-defense mechanisms. The stomach's highly acidic environment is one of the most powerful of these, efficiently destroying any viable microbes before they can enter the small intestine.

Pancreatic enzymes, bile, and other intestinal secretions are also beneficial in killing unwanted microbes. The major assumption is that a healthy bowel will take care of removing any other potentially harmful bacteria or toxic agents.

However, adherents of colonic cleansing believe that the bowel needs help to accomplish this crucial task. That is where the concept of "autointoxication" comes into play.

Irritable Bowel Syndrome

Also known as IBS or spastic colon, Irritable Bowel Syndrome is diagnosed via an examination of existing symptoms and after excluding other conditions.

The syndrome is characterized by chronic abdominal pain, bloating, and a marked alteration of bowel habits, which may include alternating episodes of diarrhea and constipation.

There is no cure, and treatment is based solely on symptom relief, with dietary adjustments and psychological assistance as major management components. Stress reduction is often critical to seeing real improvement in cases of IBS.

Whipple's Disease

A rare bacterial infection, Whipple attacks the gastrointestinal system and hampers its ability to absorb fats, carbohydrates, and other nutrients.

If left untreated with antibiotics, Whipples can spread to the brain, heart, eyes, and joints. In severe cases, the condition is fatal.

Symptoms include, but are not limited to, abdominal pain and cramping (especially after meals), diarrhea, and accompanying weight loss.

The joints of the ankles, knees, and wrists may be inflamed. In addition, the patient will likely suffer from anemia with concurrent fatigue and weakness.

Little is known about the bacteria that causes Whipples. However, it is seen most commonly in Caucasian men between the ages of 40 and 60 living in North America.

The Dangers of a Toxic Colon

A lot of professionals feel like the current healthcare system is broken. The U.S. Government Accountability Office (GAO) has found that an increasing number of senior citizens in the United States are in poor health. Experts in mortality statistics note that Americans today live longer than their grandparents. Still, they also note that chronic diseases continue to be a major burden for citizens of all ages.

According to CBS News (June 2013), roughly 70% of Americans regularly utilize the services of a licensed pharmacist.

One in ten Americans takes five or more prescription medications.

The World Health Organization (WHO) reported in 2011 that Americans have the highest healthcare costs but only the 33rd highest life expectancy.

Traditional medical practice is not geared toward providing patients with permanent healing. In its place, the pharmaceutical industry develops drugs to alleviate disease symptoms and increase profits. According to the CDC, the pharmaceutical industry in the United States earned $234.1 billion in 2008.

However, Alberto Lodola and Jeanne Stadler ("Pharmaceutical Toxicology in Practice") state that many medicines doctors prescribe for health management are harmful and toxic.

Dangers Posed by a Toxic Colon

There are three main entry points for toxins into the human body:

The human body may absorb toxins through the skin if it comes into contact with them.

Taking in a pathogen through the lungs is a surefire way to get sick.

When something is consumed or ingested, the toxin enters the digestive system and, from there, the bloodstream.

According to the doctors and naturopathic physicians at Bastyr University, roughly 90% of all toxins enter the body through the digestive tract. Therefore, the state of one's colon indicates one's general health and well-being.

The digestive system is the foundation of good health. However, the severity of the pain brought on by conditions like bloating, acne, headaches, leaky gut syndrome, food allergies and intolerances, flatulence, and constipation varies greatly.

The symptoms of a toxic colon can range from uncomfortable to fatal. Toxic megacolon is a complication of bowel disorders that can sometimes be fatal, as The New York Times reports. Warning signs of underlying colon disease may remain untreated until a crisis results. Avoiding this life-threatening condition requires prompt medical attention.

Slow Colon and Digestive System

According to a naturopath, Dr. Edward Group III ("Health Begins In The Colon"), people must regularly clean their colons to regain health or stay healthy. A toxic colon can result from a lack of routine cleansing. In addition, digestive residue causes the individual to have fewer bowel movements. Some people have only two bowel movements per week, and their doctors consider this normal. Dr. Group says that healthy individuals have two or more daily bowel movements.

Frequent bowel movements reduce many issues related to the development of a toxic colon, including the fermentation and putrefaction of digestive waste products in the body. However, left untreated, the sluggish digestive system may allow toxic wastes to leak into other parts of the body or the bloodstream. This leakage is frequently referred to as "leaky gut syndrome."

Physical Symptoms of a Slow, Toxic Colon

Many painful physical symptoms are associated with colon toxicity. Some of the most common symptoms include:

Constipation. The buildup of metabolic waste and toxins in the colon does not happen overnight. After years of waste accumulation, the sufferer's "colonic transit time" decreases. In other words, the individual has fewer bowel movements or suffers pain when trying to eliminate feces. According to the Centers for Disease Control, one in five Americans suffers from constipation or digestive problems .

Fatigue. A weakened immune system caused by a sluggish or toxic colon almost always causes the sufferer to feel extremely tired. Yeast or parasites in the body consume nutrients. In some cases, the individual may develop chronic fatigue syndrome. Naturopathic physicians often attribute yeast overgrowth (candidiasis) to a toxic colon condition. By removing dietary sugars and glutens and consuming fresh juices, raw fruits, and vegetables, periodic colon cleanses, as recommended by a medical provider, can remove colon residue and kill destructive yeast.

Flatulence. Gastritis may result from a congested, toxic colon. Inflammation of the stomach lining causes discomfort and lots of flatulence. In addition, the overgrowth of yeast, parasites, and toxins in the colon may enter the colon. When parasites, yeast, and fungi invade cells and organs, the body's immune system is progressively weakened.

Food allergies. The author of "What You Don't Know May Be Killing You" (Donald Colbert, 2013) says cooked and highly processed foods drain metabolic enzymes. Low enzyme levels allow undigested residues to remain too long in the large intestine. When these wastes are not excreted, "excessive toxic waste" in the colon results in food allergies and chronic or degenerative diseases. For these reasons, colon cleansing and a diet of natural, preferably organic, and raw foods is sometimes prescribed by a health care provider.

Headaches. Candida, parasites, toxins, and other fungi growing in a toxic colon cause migraines and other headaches, says Bruce Semon, M.D., Ph.D., of the Wisconsin Institute of Nutrition.

People may also suffer from "impaction," or a colon, without knowing it. Presenting symptoms, like headaches, are not always directly linked to digestive issues. Instead, fecal or mucous deposits stick to the colon walls, making it difficult for the highly muscular colon to contract and move. As a result, yeast, toxins, and even parasites may increase in the colon.

Colonics and Enemas

The colon is a human sewer pipe that needs a good cleaning from time to time. For best results, have a professional colonic done weekly. Enemas: Blend one raw garlic clove and three tablespoons of apple cider vinegar with a cup of water. Add the mixture to a quart enema bag. Hang the enema bag using a self-sticking plastic hook from your local hardware store, and place it about 15 inches above the top of the bathtub.

The most convenient time to do an enema is after a bowel movement. Lie on your back in the tub in a knees-to-chest position. Allow the mixture to flow into the colon until it feels full. The enema solution need not be retained. Release and refill the colon until the enema bag is empty. Use bleach to clean the tub and shower when done.

Check your Yellow Pages phone directory for colonic irrigation services. A good colonic removes waste matter that is toxic to the body. It gives you a fresh start. Colonics combined with the use of raw or cultured foods can help prevent many intestinal problems (colitis, Crohn's, etc.) and many more elsewhere in the body, including atopic dermatitis, sinusitis, excess mucus in the sinuses and lungs, COPD, hypertension, heart disease, cancer, asthma, bronchitis, arthritis, and rheumatism.

Chapter 2: What is Colon Cancer?

Cancer that begins in the colon is called colon cancer, and cancer that begins in the rectum is called rectal cancer. Cancer affecting either of these organs may also be called colorectal cancer. Colorectal cancer is cancer of the colon and rectum, two parts of the digestive system, also known as the large intestine.

The long tube that assists in moving digested food to your rectum and out of your body.

Colon cancer develops when cells grow and divide uncontrollably, just like all other types of cancer. Your body's cells are all constantly dividing, growing, and dying. Your body maintains its health and functionality in this manner.

When you have colon cancer, the cells that line your colon and rectum continue to grow and divide even though they should be dying. These cancerous cells could have originated from colon polyps. Healthcare professionals can find precancerous polyps through screening tests before they develop into cancerous tumors.

Undiagnosed or untreated colon cancer increases the risk of spreading to other parts of your body. Layers of mucous membrane, tissue, and muscle make up your intestinal wall. The mucosa, the colon's innermost lining, is where colon cancer first manifests itself.

It comprises cells that produce and secrete fluids, including mucus. These cells have the potential to alter or mutate and produce a colon polyp. As a result, colon polyps could develop into cancer in the future. (On average, a colon polyp develops cancer after around ten years.) The cancer spreads through a layer of tissue, muscle, and the outer layer of your colon if it is not discovered and treated.

Your lymph nodes or blood vessels may allow the colon cancer to spread to other parts of your body.

What are the Risk Ractors?

Smoking: Smoking and using tobacco products, and even e-cigarettes, can raise your risk of colon cancer.

Alcohol abuse: Generally, men should limit their daily intake of alcoholic beverages to two servings. One serving of alcoholic beverages per day is recommended for women.

Even occasional drinking can raise your risk of getting cancer. So, is it worth it?

Being overweight: Consuming foods heavy in fat and calories can make you gain weight and raise your risk of developing colon cancer. Avoiding or minimizing a diet high in processed meat, such as bacon, sausage, luncheon meat, and red meat, is best. Not working out: Engaging in any exercise may lower your risk of acquiring colon cancer.

Certain medical conditions could also put one at risk of colon cancer; these include:

Family history of colon and other cancers: If a close relative has colon cancer, your risk of getting the disease may be enhanced. Your biological parents, siblings, and kids are considered close family members.

If any biological family member had colon cancer before age 45, your risk might be increased.

Inflammation of the bowels: If you have inflammatory bowel disease that affects a significant portion of your colon and lasts longer than seven years, the risk increases.

A family history of polyps: Your chance of developing colon cancer may be higher if a parent, sibling, or child has an advanced polyp. A large polyp could be an advanced polyp. When examining a polyp under a microscope, medical pathologists may label it as "progressed" if they notice certain alterations that indicate the polyp may contain malignant cells.

Symptoms of Colon Cancer

Colon cancer can exist without displaying any symptoms. Therefore, even if you experience symptoms, you might not be able to tell if physical changes are indications of colon cancer. This is true because some symptoms of colon cancer are also present in other, less serious diseases. The following are typical signs:

Blood in your stool or on it: If you observe blood in the toilet after you defecate or wipe, or if your poop appears dark or brilliant red, consult a healthcare professional. It's crucial to remember that blood in your stool does not indicate colon cancer. The appearance of your excrement might also be affected by other conditions, such as hemorrhoids and anal tears.

Consistent changes in your bowel habits: A sufferer may experience chronic constipation, diarrhea, or the feeling that you need to poop even after using the restroom, as well as severe belly (abdominal) pain. Consult a healthcare professional if you experience severe stomach pain without a known cause.

Bloating of the stomach: An unusual stomach swelling accompanied by pains. Like stomach pain, many things can give you a bloated feeling. If you have a bloated stomach that persists for more than a week, consult a doctor.

Unexpected weight loss: A significant decline in body weight occurs when you are not actively attempting to lose weight.

Risk Factors for Colorectal Cancer

There are several risk factors for developing colorectal cancer. Having one or more of these risk factors does not guarantee that a person will develop colorectal cancer; it just increases the chances. While you cannot change your medical history, genetics, or age, you can impact your future medical history. Getting appropriate screenings and developing a healthy lifestyle can increase your odds of staying healthy for longer.

Don't let the price of testing keep you from getting the care you need. Medicare covers colorectal cancer screening and will pay part or all of the cost of a fecal occult blood test, flexible sigmoidoscopy, barium enema, or colonoscopy. If fees are a concern, then talk to your doctor or local hospital about possible sliding-scale fees based on your income.

Women are just as likely as men to develop colorectal cancer, but age is a risk factor. The older you get, the more likely you are to develop colorectal cancer. Once you hit forty years old, your cancer risk increases, especially after fifty. In some cases, it can occur in teenagers and other young adults.

For some people, seeking the advice of a genetic counselor may be worthwhile. Medical researchers have learned that changes in specific genes may raise the risk of colorectal cancer. So if there are several cases of colorectal cancer in your family, you may find it helpful to talk with a genetic counselor.

Medical researchers propose that your diet may place you at a higher risk for colorectal cancer. For example, diets high in fat and calories and low in fiber may pose a higher risk. In addition, your family's genetics may influence how likely you are to develop colorectal cancer. For example, suppose you are a close relative of someone who has had colorectal cancer or another chronic digestive condition. In that case, you may have a higher-than-average risk of developing colorectal cancer.

Your own medical history impacts your likelihood of getting colorectal cancer. Women with a history of cancer in the ovary, uterus, or breast may have a slightly higher chance of developing colorectal cancer. If a person has already had colorectal cancer, then they are at a higher risk of developing the disease a second time.

Symptoms of Colorectal Cancer

Many cases of colorectal cancer have no symptoms. That's why annual screening is so important. However, if you have these symptoms and either have not yet been tested or it has been longer than a year since you were tested, then contact your physician:

Frequent gas pains

- Blood in or on the stool
- Diarrhea or constipation
- A feeling that the bowel has not emptied completely
- Blood in the stool or rectal bleeding
- Persistent change in bowel habits
- Change in the shape of the stool (such as pencil-thin feces or the presence of black, tar-like stool)
- Pain in the abdomen or rectum
- Cramping
- A frequent feeling of fullness in the rectum
- Frequent false urges to defecate
- Persistent or alternating bouts of constipation or diarrhea
- Weakness and fatigue
- Weight loss and loss of appetite
- Soilage
- Protrusion from the anal opening
- Ulcer near the anus

Screening for Colorectal Cancer

One of the major causes of cancer-related mortality in the United States is colorectal cancer, says the American Cancer Society. The good news is that a full recovery is usually possible after an early diagnosis. The most treatable stage of colon cancer is the asymptomatic stage, which can be diagnosed with screening. The American Cancer Society recommends that everyone over the age of 50 undergo a colorectal cancer screening. Tests for colon cancer screening include:

Small amounts of blood in the stool can be detected with a yearly fecal occult blood test.

Every five to seven years, a person should have a flexible colonoscopy to check for colorectal cancer.

Let's pretend for a second that a colonoscopy is out of the question. A double contrast barium enema (DCBE), a series of X-rays of the colon and rectum, is a good alternative in such cases. In order to see the patient's colon and rectum on X-rays, the patient is given a barium-containing enema solution.

The doctor does a digital rectal exam (DRE) once a year by inserting a gloved finger into the rectum while it is lubricated to check for any abnormalities.

High-risk people of any age with a history of cancer, a strong family history of the disease, or a predisposing chronic digestive condition like inflammatory bowel disease should have a colonoscopy as often as their doctor prescribes.

Chapter 3: Understanding Colorectal Cancer

Colorectal cancer, also called colon cancer or large bowel cancer, is the third most common cancer in the United States. Colon cancer symptoms may include a change in bowel habits or bleeding, but usually, colon cancer strikes without symptoms. Understand your risks and how your doctor can identify polyps before your life is at risk. New research seems to come out weekly about what you should or shouldn't be eating, drinking, or doing to prevent it. Learn what you can do to lower your risk.

Colorectal Polyps

Colorectal cancer causes an estimated 65,000 deaths yearly and is the second most common cancer killer in the United States. With 158,000 new cases of colorectal cancer diagnosed annually, men and women are equally at risk for this type of cancer.

All colon cancers begin as polyps. Polyps are small, abnormal growths that form on the colon's wall. If left untreated, polyps may become cancerous over time. However, if polyps are identified and removed at an early stage, they do not have the opportunity to become cancerous.

Risks of Diverticulosis

Diverticulosis is a disorder of the colon. A healthy colon is sturdy and unruffled. However, diverticulosis causes the walls to be weakened in specific places. This causes the colon to protrude in tiny pouches at the weak points. Consider a tire where the inner tube has poked through a crack. Each little bag is about the size of a big pea.

It wasn't until the early 1900s that the disease made its way to the forefront of public consciousness in the United States. The NDDIC notes an increase in digestive disorders around the same time that processed foods became commonplace in the American diet. Refined, low-fiber flour is a common ingredient in processed foods. Refined flour lacks the beneficial fibers and proteins found in wheat bran, making it inferior to whole-wheat flour.

A diverticulum is a bag in the colon that only contains one diverticulum. Although diverticulosis can manifest itself anywhere along the length of the colon, the majority of cases show up on the left side. The sigmoid colon is the section of the colon that is both the narrowest and has the highest intramural pressure.

Discovering Polyps

As many as 80 percent of people with diverticulosis never realize they have it. It is a very common disorder in people over sixty. More than half of all people between the ages of sixty and eighty have diverticulosis, and nearly everyone over the age of eighty has the condition.

Diverticulosis can be difficult to diagnose because it usually causes no symptoms. It is usually discovered during an intestinal examination. Tests like barium enema X-rays, flexible sigmoidoscopy, or colonoscopy examinations can all be helpful diagnostic tools.

Diverticulitis Risks

Diverticulosis is a condition characterized by the formation of pouches on the colon lining. When the pouches become inflamed and infected, the condition is known as diverticulitis. Stool contains bacteria that can cause an infection if it becomes trapped in a pouch. Left lower abdominal pain or soreness may be a sign of diverticulitis.

Fever, nausea, vomiting, chills, cramps, and constipation are all possible symptoms of infection. The severity of the symptoms will depend on the nature of the illness and any complications that have developed. Bleeding, infections, rips, and intestinal obstructions are among the potential complications of diverticulitis.

Patients at high risk for colon polyps, which are precursors to colon cancer, can reduce their polyp count by taking aspirin daily, according to studies published in the New England Journal of Medicine. See your doctor about making aspirin part of your regular routine.

Antibiotic treatment is the standard for diverticulitis. When the symptoms of diverticulitis are mild, they can usually be treated with antibiotics taken by mouth. Antibiotics like doxycycline (Vibramycin), amoxicillin (Ambien), and ciprofloxacin (Cipro), to name a few, are often prescribed (Vibramycin). Patients suffering from an acute bout of diverticulitis should stick to liquid diets or foods low in fiber. Some people with severe cases of diverticulitis, characterized by high fever and pain, require hospitalization and intravenous antibiotics.

Diverticulosis Causes and Treatment

Constipation appears to be the culprit for the condition. When you are constipated, the muscles strain to move too-hard stool. That strain is the main cause of increased pressure in the colon. This excess pressure might cause the weak spots in the colon to bulge out. Other risk factors include:

- Diet low in fiber content or high in fat

- High intake of meat and red meat
- Increasing age
- Constipation
- Connective tissue disorders that may cause weakness in the colon wall

Diverticulitis Treatment

Once diverticula have formed, there is no way to reverse the process. The pouches are there for the rest of your life. In addition, some people find that eating nuts and seeds during an attack of diverticulitis can irritate the inflamed intestinal lining.

When to Seek Medical Care

Seek medical attention if you have these symptoms:

- Persistent abdominal pain
- Persistent unexplained fevers
- Persistent diarrhea
- Persistent vomiting
- A urinary tract infection that won't go away

Any time you have bleeding from your rectum, you should immediately see your health care provider. This is true even if the bleeding stops on its own. Bleeding may be a sign of diverticulitis or other serious diseases. If there is a lot of blood or a steady flow of blood, go to a hospital emergency department immediately.

During diverticulitis attacks, many doctors suggest mild pain medication and bowel rest. Bowel rest usually involves two to three days of clear fluids (no food), so your colon may heal without working.

Preventing Diverticulitis

Once you have had diverticulitis, your odds are high. It will return. To reduce the odds of diverticula becoming inflamed or infected, follow the same recommendations to prevent constipation.

For chronic constipation, try one of these variations of pudding power: In a blender, blend 1 cup of crushed 100 percent bran flakes with 1½ cups of canned pears in their juice. You can substitute the pears with 1 cup of applesauce and ½ cup of prune juice. To take the pudding, drink an 8-ounce glass of warm water, followed by a tablespoon of pudding powder a day for the first week, two tablespoons a day for the second week, and so on, up to five tablespoons a day.

Eat a high-fiber diet, drink plenty of fluids, and exercise regularly. Aim for 38 grams of fiber per day for men and 25 grams per day for women.

Living with IBS

Irritable bowel syndrome affects the large intestine and causes many problems, including bloating, abdominal cramping, diarrhea, and constipation. It occurs when the intestines squeeze too hard or not hard enough, causing food to move too quickly or too slowly through the intestines. It is also known as functional bowel syndrome, irritable colon, spastic bowel, and spastic colon. IBS is not a disease—it's a functional disorder—and it's characterized as a brain-gut dysfunction.

IBS Sufferers

More than 20 percent of Americans suffer from IBS, which affects more women (75 percent) than men. This is because women may have more frequent symptoms during their menstrual periods.

Irritable bowel syndrome (IBS) does not have to rule your life. Many people have symptoms mild enough not to disrupt their lives. However, for about a fourth of people diagnosed with IBS, work, school, and other activities are sometimes disrupted. At times, eating a specific type of food may trigger symptoms. For others, physical and emotional factors play a role, and stressful events may affect their symptoms.

Symptoms of IBS

IBS symptoms vary from person to person and can vary in severity and duration among individuals. Typical symptoms include:

- Diarrhea
- Constipation
- Bloating
- Excess gas
- Abdominal pain
- Nausea
- Back pain

It's Not All in Your Head

One of the most common misconceptions about IBS is that it is purely a psychological problem. It isn't. It is a real physiological condition that can be mild, irritating, excruciating, and life-changing.

However, IBS is made worse by stress. Stress can aggravate all kinds of medical conditions. For example, asthmatics can suffer from an asthma attack when stressed, and IBS patients can have an IBS attack. That doesn't mean that IBS is caused by stress any more than asthma is caused by stress.

Get a Diagnosis

The cause of irritable bowel syndrome isn't known, and getting a diagnosis can be difficult. IBS patients see an average of three physicians over three years before receiving a diagnosis. It used to be thought of as a diagnosis of exclusion. That is, it was diagnosed by ruling out everything else first. If nothing's left, it must be IBS. That is no longer true.

Because IBS is not a disease, diagnosis depends partly on determining whether or not your symptoms match those that have been medically established as definitive of IBS.

With the Rome criteria, you are believed to have IBS if abdominal pain or discomfort is continuous or comes and goes for a total of at least twelve weeks during the year. Two of the three following conditions occur:

- Pain is relieved by having a bowel movement
- The frequency of bowel movements changes
- The stools' appearance or form changes
- Mistaken Identity—When It's Not IBS

Making a diagnosis of IBS can be difficult, and it is necessary to rule out other potential digestive health concerns. It can be helpful to know that these symptoms are not typical of IBS: pain or diarrhea that often awakens or interferes with sleep, blood in your stool (visible or occult), weight loss, or fever.

People with irritable bowel syndrome are statistically more likely to have upper GI problems (like GERD or reflux). However, they are not more likely to develop colon cancer.

Where did the Rome criteria for irritable bowel syndrome originate?

At the 13th International Congress of Gastroenterology in Rome, Italy, in 1988, a group of physicians developed a system to classify functional gastrointestinal disorders based on clinical symptoms. Known as the Rome criteria, the guidelines outline symptoms and apply parameters such as frequency and duration to make possible a more accurate diagnosis of IBS and other digestive disorders.

IBS Self-Care

Irritable bowel syndrome (IBS) patients have found these suggestions helpful:

Throw out anything that contains carrageenan (this includes soy milk and ice cream).

Probiotics, which contain beneficial bacteria, should be taken at mealtimes in order to maintain gastrointestinal health.

Diarrhea treatment with carob powder (mix a tablespoon with applesauce and honey). This medicine, when used on occasion, can calm an aggravated digestive tract. If you're experiencing cramping or soreness in your abdomen, peppermint oil may also help. Take one or two enteric-coated capsules, thrice daily, 15 to30 minutes before eating.

Powdered slippery elm might help. One teaspoon of the powder, one teaspoon of sugar, and two cups of boiling water can be made into a comforting gruel. One or two cups per day, stirred thoroughly, with cinnamon added for flavor.

Consume 500 milligrams to 1 gram of turmeric daily. It's a potent anti-inflammatory medication that can help with microscopic inflammation in the stomach, which is another potential cause of IBS.

Consider Dietary Changes

Everyone with IBS responds differently to food, so there is no one-size-fits-all diet that can assist. It's best to avoid eating anything that's particularly high in fat, insoluble fiber, caffeine, coffee (even decaf), carbonation, or alcohol. Why? The gastrocolic reflex can be triggered violently by certain types of food because they are either GI stimulants or irritants. Pain, constipation or diarrhea, gas, and bloating are all symptoms of irritated colon muscles that these substances might cause.

Avoiding dairy is often recommended for those who suffer from IBS. Many people experience discomfort after consuming dairy products, even if they are not lactose intolerant. Replace your regular milk with rice milk. Most IBS sufferers should eat a low-fat, high-protein diet and avoid these items:

- Alcohol
- Caffeine found in coffee, tea, many carbonated drinks, and chocolate
- Nicotine from smoking or chewing tobacco
- Dairy products that contain lactose (milk sugar), such as milk, cheese, and sour cream
- Spicy foods, including salsas or many ethnic foods that use chile peppers
- Foods high in acid, such as citrus fruit

- Foods high in fat, including bacon, sausage, butter, oils, and anything deep-fried
- Sorbitol and xylitol, artificial sweeteners found in some sugarless candies and chewing gum

Dietary Downfalls

Many people with IBS find it helpful to keep meals low in fat and high in carbohydrates. Carbohydrates include bread, pasta, rice, fruits, vegetables, and cereals. Some foods that you will be able to tolerate include:

Bread and Grains

- Whole-wheat flour, whole-wheat bread, whole-wheat cereal
- Wheat bran, whole grains, whole-grain bread, whole-grain cereals
- Granola, muesli, seeds, and nuts
- Popcorn
- Beans and lentils

Fruit

- Berries, grapes, raisins, and cherries
- Pineapples, peaches, nectarines, apricots, and pears with skins
- Rhubarb
- Melons
- Oranges, grapefruits, lemons, limes
- Dates and prunes

Vegetables

- Greens (spinach, lettuce, kale, mesclun, collards, arugula, watercress, and so on)
- Whole peas, snow peas, snap peas, pea pods
- Green beans, kernel corn
- Bell peppers (roasted and peeled. They're safer)
- Eggplant (peeled and seeded, it's much safer)
- Celery, onions, shallots, leeks, scallions, garlic
- Cabbage, bok choy, Brussels sprouts
- Broccoli, cauliflower

Take Control of Your Colon Health

You have a great deal of power to improve your health. Maintain a healthy weight, talk to a genetic counselor, don't smoke, and exercise. In addition, reducing your radiation exposure can be one more step toward protecting your colon.

Eating for Colon Health

You cannot prevent cancer by eating certain things, but scientists believe what you choose to eat (and avoid) can decrease your likelihood of developing cancer. The following recipes were developed using the latest in colorectal research and are all low-fat and high-fiber.

Listen to Your Body

You aren't supposed to hurt. Digestive problems are not normal. Don't brush off the uncomfortable signals your body is trying to give you. If something doesn't feel right, get it checked out.

Is it okay to eat red meat if I'm concerned about colon cancer?

Go for the fish instead. In a major study of 478,000 people, those who ate six ounces of red and processed meat daily were one-third more likely to have colon cancer than those who ate less than one ounce per day.

Regular Checkups

The facts are simple. You could have colon cancer or a precancerous condition and not know it. While researchers believe diet, exercise, genetics, and lifestyle play a role in colon health, even people who do all the right things get cancer. If you avoid getting tests and exams done regularly, you are taking a risk with your health.

The Colon and the pH factor

PH represents the "potential Hydrogen" absorbing capacity of a substance. A pH of "0" means a substance is as acidic (i.e., sulfuric acid) as it can get and will absorb no more hydrogen atoms. At a pH of 13, a substance can absorb lots of hydrogen ions (i.e., ammonia is alkaline). The digestive process requires hydrochloric acid in the stomach but needs a neutral or slightly alkaline pH in the small intestines. When the food reaches the large intestines, the pH drops to around 6 in healthy individuals.

Friendly acid-producing bacteria help to move colonic pH (down) in an acidic direction. When the pH of the colon is alkaline (above 7.0), all kinds of unwanted pathogens, from viruses to fungus to bacteria, set up housekeeping and can cause havoc with your immune system by producing toxins and harmful chemicals that burden the liver, kidneys, and the immune system.

Bech K et al. (18) found that in measuring the pH of the feces,"significantly higher pH values ..... were found in patients with cancer than in normal individuals." He wrote, "These results support the performance of intervention trials with lowering the pH of the colon with the object of cancer prophylaxis...."

Research published in the Journal of AIDS, PNAS, and Nature's Medicine has found that up to 86% of all HIV lives in the intestines. If the pH of the colon is higher than 6.0, cell-free HIV can infect CD4 cells and continue replicating, but when the pH is less than 6.0, cell-free HIV permanently loses its ability to infect new cells (20).

Anecdotal reports from persons with Chronic Fatigue Syndrome (CFS), cancer, and candidiasis who have had stool samples analyzed report the following:

High pH values are usually in the 7.0 - 9.0 range.

Little or no acidophilus was found in the stools.

Low butyrate levels indicate low bifidobacteria counts.

High levels of candida Albicans and other unfriendly flora.

These abnormal values are often associated with food allergies, leaky gut syndrome, and a weak intestinal wall. People with CFIDS, candidiasis, and severe food allergies frequently find that the only foods they can tolerate are vegetables and proteins. Persons with CFIDS, candidiasis, hepatitis, and cancer who are doing poorly always report stools that sink (in the toilet bowl) and sometimes have a small diameter, indicating inflammation in the intestines.

Diet for a Healthy Colon

Our colon is what we eat. No matter what we consume, it all travels through our body and eventually reaches our colon. As a result, the majority of diseases affecting the colon are caused by our diet. If we want our colon to stay healthy, we must ensure that only healthy food reaches it.

Consume micro flora-fortified products

Yogurt and fermented milk fortified with Lactobacilli are readily available in grocery stores. These encourage good bacteria to grow in the colon. Lacto bacteria also prevent bile from converting into bile acid.

Drink Milk

Some studies indicate that calcium and vitamin D might decrease the chances of developing colorectal cancer. A word of caution, though: one can also go overboard with calcium. The best is to keep calcium around 1,000-1,300 milligrams a day. You can meet this requirement by drinking around three 8-ounces glasses of low-fat or fat-free milk daily. In addition, you can supplement calcium from other sources, such as green leafy vegetables.

Fish

To maintain a healthy colon, replace your red meat consumption with fish. It's always a good choice.

Increase Fiber Intake

There is never too much fiber for the colon. A high-fiber diet can even make a couple of dietary wrongs right. Fiber ensures you are never constipated and always on time for your daily excretion. Fiber also keeps you away from hemorrhoids. An adult's recommended daily amount of fiber is 25-35 grams.

The best part about fiber is that it comes in various forms. There are plenty of fiber-rich vegetables and fruits to choose from: cooked artichokes, broccoli, corn, peas, oranges, apples, pears, and raspberries. Whole grains and legumes also have high fiber content.

Start Using a Variety of Whole Grains

Whole grains contain vital nutrients, such as vitamins, minerals, antioxidants, and phytochemicals, which are very colon-friendly. According to the Dietary Guidelines for Americans, half of your daily grain consumption should come from whole grains. Another suggestion is to include a variety of grains in the diet. For example, include grains such as barley, brown rice, quinoa, and oatmeal in your daily consumption.

Brown rice also contains short-chain fatty acids that inhibit the growth of cancerous cells.

Water

Fiber absorbs water. Therefore, if you increase your fiber intake, increase your water consumption. Drinking eight glasses of water every day is an absolute must.

Don'ts

Limited Red Meat Consumption and Steering Sway from Processed Meat

The American Cancer Society reports that even a once-a-day diet of 100 grams of red meat or 50 grams of processed meat can increase the risk of colon cancer by 15% to 20%. That means it's not good for your colon to eat hamburgers, sausages, or hotdogs every day. As long as you stick to sensible serving sizes, eating red meat is completely OK. You can safely have up to several 4-ounce portions of red meat per week. Avoid processed meats whenever possible.

Control Your Sugar Consumption

One of the reasons behind many colon-related diseases like ulcerative colitis and Crohn's disease is a diet high in sugar and low in fiber.

Consuming foods high in sugar can ultimately lead to weight gain and obesity. In addition, the National Cancer Institute has linked obesity with an increased risk of colon cancer.

Chapter 4: Why Gut Health is Important

The gastrointestinal tract, also known as the gut, is extremely important to your overall health. It accounts for 70% of your immunity. It is the body's largest endocrine organ and the second brain. It produces vitamins, excretes waste, and regulates your hormones.

Several studies have also found links between the digestive tract and human health. One of these notable connections is the presence of millions of bacteria in your gut and your ability to protect yourself from diseases. When your gut contains more bad bacteria than good bacteria, your body's ability to detoxify and eliminate harmful substances decreases. In contrast, having more good bacteria makes your body more resistant to disease.

Toxins are also prevented from entering your bloodstream by the environment of your intestinal tract. Your body is protected from pathogens by the cellular lining and its chemical barriers. Any change in these components predisposes you to cancer, depression, and obesity.

Weakening and increased permeability of the intestinal walls, also known as leaky gut syndrome, can result in various health problems. Toxins and waste products leak through the porous walls, triggering an immune system reaction. It has been linked to food allergies, arthritis, autism, and learning disabilities.

Aside from immunity, your gut plays an important role in your mental health. This is because your gut has a nervous system that communicates with your brain. This is also known as your enteric nervous system, which is responsible for your upset stomach when you're angry or tense. It's also why, when you're nervous, you get butterflies in your stomach.

The link between your gut and your brain causes anxiety and depression. Serotonin, in particular, plays a significant role in why these mental conditions occur in people. Serotonin is a neurotransmitter that plays a role in various brain functions. It has an impact on your mood, sleep, and appetite. Although it is more associated with mental functions, your gut contains and produces a large amount of serotonin. Your mental health may suffer if your body's requirement for this neurotransmitter is not met or if your gut is not healthy enough to produce serotonin.

Our digestive tract is responsible for both what we eat and excrete. Therefore, we will not be able to receive the nutrients we require for optimal health if it fails to break down the food we put in our mouths. On that note, if the gut does not eliminate toxins and they build up inside the body, the system becomes toxic, and we become ill.

The significance of gut health is obvious. On the other hand, keeping it in good shape is a different and more complicated story. With today's unhealthy food choices and habits, it's no surprise that more people are getting sick every day. If your health is currently suffering or you want to be healthy, you can restore it by listening to your gut. You are healthy if your gut is healthy.

Take Care About Your Gut

It appears that Hippocrates' observation that "all diseases, in a way, begin in the gut" was prescient. Inadequate gut health has been linked by scientific research to various illnesses.

Guts, in the sense of the digestive system, are something that every human being possesses. In bilaterians, it plays a role in the digestive process. Animals with bilateral symmetry can be easily identified because their bodies are split down the middle, with a left and right side and a front and back. Humans are part of this category.

The digestive process begins when food enters the mouth and travels down the gastrointestinal tract to the stomach and other digestive organs. The anus is the opening through which waste products from large bilaterian animals such as whales and pigs are expelled. The anus's main job is to regulate the elimination of waste products like feces and undigested food.

Thousands of distinct species of bacteria can be found in the digestive system. However, humans' most common types of gut bacteria fall into one of three categories. Human gut flora refers to the microbial population that lives there.

There is a vital and dynamic connection between the functions of your gut and immune system and your brain, as shown by research. Digestion-assisting gut microbes also influence satiety, body composition, and vitality. All of these factors point to one conclusion: your gut health has a major impact on your overall health, and maintaining it can aid in managing nutritional conditions and weight issues. Your gut health can even influence your mental makeup. Nutrition in Clinical Practice is the journal where you can find the study's findings.

Common Diseases of the Gut

The gut, just like any other system of the body, is also prone to various kinds of diseases. Some gut diseases are short-lived and easily treated, while others are chronic and require specific medications. Some conditions also require specific lifestyle changes, particularly in diet.

There are a lot of different conditions and disorders that are associated with the gastrointestinal tract. The following are several examples of disorders that may affect the digestive system.

Acute Diarrhea

People have different numbers of bowel movements. Some people move their bowels once a day, others more than once or only a few times a week. Normally, people move their bowels around three times a day and three times a week with normal, solid stools. It is called diarrhea when the stools are passed more than three times a day and are loose and watery.

The symptoms of diarrhea may suddenly occur and clear up within 5 to 10 days. An infection of the intestines, called gastroenteritis, commonly causes it. Intestinal infections usually occur in infants and young children because of their immature immune systems. Infant diarrhea is usually caused by rotavirus.

Acute diarrhea may also be caused by bacteria (through food poisoning), such as Campylobacter and Salmonella. Food poisoning may happen when bacteria contaminate food, water, eggs, or poultry. It may also be acquired from an infected but asymptomatic person who handles food.

Travelers are also more prone to acute diarrhea. Escherichia coli commonly causes it. E. coli releases enterotoxins in the gut, which may encourage gut secretions.

Alcohol intake, drugs, anxiety attacks, and antibiotics may cause acute diarrhea. Acute diarrhea may clear up within a few days. But if it persists for more than a few days, medical intervention may be required.

Celiac Disease

Celiac disease is a condition that is caused by a hypersensitivity to a type of protein called gluten. In this condition, gluten may irritate the lining of the small intestines. It is believed to affect only 1% of people and usually remains undiagnosed and asymptomatic.

Symptoms of celiac disease may include vomiting, diarrhea, failure to gain weight, weight loss, mouth sores, and abdominal pain. The best treatment for celiac disease is to avoid gluten-containing foods.

It is a good thing that gluten is not necessary for the body. Thus, it can be easily replaced in the diet through proper planning and preparation of meals. In addition, a visit to the doctor may help in the proper diagnosis of celiac disease.

Constipation

Constipation is a condition that is more of a symptom than an illness in and of itself. It is characterized by difficulty passing stools. Constipated people may pass hard, pellet-like stools, have fewer bowel movements (fewer than three times per week), and strain during bowel motions.

Constipation can be caused by various factors, including a lack of activity, a diet low in fruits, vegetables, and fiber, a rapid lifestyle change, and neglecting the urge to pass stools. In addition, constipation, as well as being overweight or underweight, can be caused by increased stress.

Treatment for constipation focuses on addressing the causes listed above. It is easily treatable. It rarely causes long-term issues.

Crohn's Disease

Crohn's disease is a condition that is characterized by inflammation in the gut. It is associated with one of the two conditions, such as Ulcerative Colitis and Inflammatory Bowel Disease. It is characterized by symptoms that include diarrhea, pain, ulcers, loss of appetite, and fatigue.

Crohn's disease may affect any area of the gut. However, it normally affects the top of the large intestines or the bottom of the small intestines (lower part of the gut). It is prevalent in people aged 15 to 40. However, it only affects 1 in 650 people.

The cause of this disease is not yet known. But it is believed to be linked with genetics. One in five people with Crohn's disease has a family member with the same condition.

Smokers are more likely to develop this disease, although both men and women have equal chances of being affected by it. It is not likely to be caused by specific dietary patterns.

The treatment of Crohn's disease primarily focuses on reducing the inflammation of the intestines. Most cases of this disease require surgery. However, some cases can be treated through drug therapy or dietary changes.

Diarrhea

Diarrhea is a condition that causes feces to become loose, watery, and frequent. It is also possible to experience stomach aches, which may subside after passing stools. There are two types of diarrhea: chronic (long-term) and acute (short-term).

Occasionally, acute diarrhea is caused by an infection or a virus. It can be contracted through contaminated food or spread from person to person. Excessive alcohol use, certain medications, or stress can also cause it. Acute diarrhea can be treated with over-the-counter medications, good hygiene, and plenty of fluids. This could improve in a few days.

Irritable Bowel Syndrome is the most common cause of chronic diarrhea. It is, however, linked to hormonal fluctuations, drugs, and Inflammatory Bowel Disease. Chronic diarrhea is defined as diarrhea that lasts two weeks or more. Therefore, seeing a doctor to correctly diagnose the underlying reason and provide the required medical treatment is critical.

Gallstones

Gallstones are bile crystals that grow in the bile duct or gall bladder. Normally, the liver produces bile, which is finally deposited in the gallbladder. It is made up of various compounds, but if there are too many of them, it might form gallstones.

Gallstones can range in size from a grain of sand to a golf ball. These frequently contain cholesterol, a chemical that is naturally present in bile. It is more prevalent in older people and women. It is frequently asymptomatic. Symptoms such as stomach pain may emerge only if the gallstones travel to the bile duct. Therefore, asymptomatic gallstones should be left alone. On the other hand, gallstones that cause severe pain can be removed with keyhole surgery.

Heartburn (acid reflux)

The food we eat passes from the mouth through the stomach. The food we consume moves in only one direction. However, in the case of acid reflux, the food travels back up into the esophagus. It is called reflux or regurgitation. This is not the same as vomiting, which is a violent reaction. Reflux can happen without the person even realizing it.

Reflux is controlled by a muscle ring at the esophagus's lower end. While eating, the muscle ring relaxes and then tightens after eating. But then, it could sag, and reflux may occur. However, there is no clear reason for the sagging of the muscle ring of the esophagus.

Reflux symptoms are characterized by a burning sensation in the chest and may be called heartburn. Repeated reflux may lead to a condition called esophagitis. It is the scratching and swelling of the lining of the esophagus.

Hemorrhoids or piles

A hemorrhoid is a condition characterized by inflammation of the blood vessels in the anus and rectum. It is very common and affects approximately 50% of the population at some point in their lives.

There are two different types of hemorrhoids: internal and external hemorrhoids. Internal hemorrhoids occur inside the rectum. External hemorrhoids occur outside the anus. It is distinguished by itching around the anus and bleeding from the affected area. Another symptom is difficulty passing stools.

It is caused by extreme pressure on the blood vessels in the rectum during difficult bowel movements, pregnancy (weight of the abdomen), and obesity (weight of the core).

The treatment of hemorrhoids focuses on addressing the symptoms, such as altering the diet by increasing fiber intake to ease bowel movement, sitting in a hot sitz bath to relieve itchiness, and taking medications.

Another common hemorrhoid treatment is a procedure called banding. It is done by securing a band around the blood vessel to decrease the blood supply. In other cases, surgery may be required to remove hemorrhoids.

Indigestion

Indigestion happens when one eats food in a rush or when one eats or drinks too much. It is a painful sensation at the top of the abdomen below the chest that occurs right after drinking or eating. It is more of a symptom than a disease, but it can be very annoying.

It rarely causes serious problems. However, if it occurs later in life, it is best to seek medical help. It is more common in people who experience gastrointestinal reflux and those who take medications for arthritis.

Esophageal and stomach cancer, pancreatic diseases, and gallstones rarely cause it. A mild case of indigestion is called non-ulcer dyspepsia.

Irritable Bowel Syndrome

IBS, or Irritable Bowel Syndrome, is a term used to describe the combination of symptoms of the disorder of the large intestine. 30% of people may experience IBS sometime in their lives. Around 1 in 10 sufferers seek medical attention. It is a distressing condition that may need medical attention and treatment.

Symptoms of IBS may include constipation, diarrhea, abdominal spasms, abdominal pain, stomach rumbling sounds, excessive farting, swelling or bloating of the abdomen, incontinence, sharp pain in the lower rectum, an urge to pass stools, and a feeling of an incomplete bowel movement.

IBS is more common in women than men, in Western countries than others, and in young people than older adults. It is linked to emotional tension, sudden changes in lifestyle, and stressful situations.

IBS has no cure, and the symptoms may vary from person to person. Therefore, the treatment may also vary from person to person, depending on the symptoms. Anti-spasmodic medications and diet changes are usual treatments for IBS. Alternative treatments may include probiotic intake, acupuncture, and homeopathy.

Ulcerative Colitis

This is a condition that is characterized by long-term inflammation of the colon. Severe inflammation of the colon may cause ulcers to develop. The inflammation is usually limited to the rectal area. On the other hand, some people may have the entire colon affected.

Symptoms of ulcerative colitis include diarrhea, abdominal pain, and rectal bleeding. It is most common in people ages 15 to 30. Men and women have equal chances of having this kind of condition.

The causes of ulcerative colitis are still unknown. Yet, it is believed that it is caused by the response of the colon to a large number of bacteria in the gut. It can be treated with medications. However, severe cases of Ulcerative Colitis may require surgery.

Habits for a Healthy Gut

One's general health and well-being may greatly benefit from maintaining good gut health. Conversely, poor gut health can undo all the hard work put into maintaining one's physical health. The digestive process begins in the gut, also called the gastrointestinal tract. It's the foundation of a happy and healthy life. Because of this, it affects how much of certain substances and nutrients the body takes in.

Lack of good gut health has been linked to problems in the nervous system, immune response, and hormone secretions. In addition, neurons (similar to those found in the brain) are abundant in the digestive tract and may impact one's emotional state. The use of the phrase "gut feelings" is blamed for this.

Food travels through the digestive system from the mouth before being expelled as solid waste through the anus. The digestion process, nutrient absorption, and waste elimination depend on the gut's proper functioning. However, gut permeability can be damaged and influenced by things like viruses, parasites, poor nutrition, alcohol consumption, caffeine consumption, NSAIDs, antibiotics, and pathogenic bacteria. The leaky gut syndrome describes this ailment.

A leaky gut is characterized by the inability of the intestinal lining to prevent small particles of undigested food from entering the bloodstream. This condition could bring on inflammation and the secretion of stress hormones. Cortisol is one such stress hormone, and others may also impair immunity. Possible side effects include accelerated skin aging, allergies, gastrointestinal distress, and unchecked weight gain.

Fortunately, despite the many threats to digestive health, some things can be done to heal the intestines. In addition, the immune system and neurotransmitter production may benefit from restoring gut health.

The first step is to clean up your diet by ditching all the junk and processed foods. This may be one of the causes of digestive distress. Alcohol, caffeine, bad cholesterol, processed foods, dairy, and gluten can all aggravate the digestive tract and should be avoided. In addition, inflammation of the intestines is a possible result of irritation.

Intestinal lining repair comes next. Healing a leaky gut may be aided by eating whole, unprocessed foods. Healing of the digestive tract can be aided by getting plenty of shut-eye. Omega-3 fatty acids, L-glutamine, vitamins A, E, and C, zinc, turmeric, aloe vera, and other things may aid gut healing.

The following are some food supplements that may help restore and maintain gut health.

High-grade fish oil: Fish oil in liquid (not capsule) form is best for gut health. It helps boost the immune system, reduce inflammation, and balance hormonal levels. However, liquid fish oil has an unpleasant taste.

L-Glutamine: This supplement helps in healing and sealing a leaky gut. It is also helpful in recovering after physical workouts.

Cinnamon: This can be added to foods to help improve digestion. It can also help lower blood sugar levels.

Probiotic supplements provide good bacteria for the gut. It may also help increase the gut's immune defenses by increasing the number of good microorganisms.

Zinc: Zinc is crucial for forming digestive enzymes. It is also beneficial for regulating hormones.

Mint: Mint has a relaxing effect on the gastrointestinal tract. It may also help soothe an upset stomach.

Alkaline or pH-balancing foods: Some examples of alkaline foods are leafy greens, such as spinach, kale, wheatgrass, broccoli, spirulina, chlorella, and parsley. These may help in keeping the stomach acid levels in order.

Prebiotics: Prebiotics are present in fermented foods. Prebiotics nourishes good bacteria by letting them flourish in a healthy environment. Some examples include sauerkraut, yogurt, kimchi, and kefir.

Another way to maintain a healthy gut is by restoring its natural flora. It can be done by introducing good bacteria, such as Bifidobacterium lactis and Lactobacillus acidophilus. In addition, good bacteria, or probiotics, can help maintain a healthy gastrointestinal tract and protect it from various illnesses.

Around 85% of good bacteria make up a healthy intestinal tract. The abundance of good bacteria inhibits the growth of bad or pathogenic bacteria. However, the balance of good and bad bacteria in the gut may be altered and affect one's health. For example, Clostridium and Salmonella (bad bacteria) can be found in the human gut. Nonetheless, it is all right if it is kept at safe levels.

The last step involves keeping hydrochloric acid, bile salts, and stomach enzymes at favorable levels to encourage proper digestion. It can be done by supplementing with organic salt and enzymes.

Chapter 5: Home remedies to Keep your Colon Healthy

Colon cleansing is not just about supplements and colon irrigation; several other aspects that occur naturally can help you clean and maintain your colon. You also don't have to go through any weird fad diets or spend days on end sitting on the toilet with cramps. What you eat has a direct impact on your colon, and maintaining a healthy diet can reduce your risk of digestive diseases and even colon cancer.

Using Water to flush Toxins

The best strategy to flush toxins out of your body is to consume water rather than pump water into your body in another manner. Because our bodies are made up of roughly 60% water, water is vital to the human body and the colon. Remember how fiber absorbs water to bulk up excrement in the colon, promoting smoother passage? Unfortunately, you can still become constipated and develop other colon-related problems if you only eat fiber and don't drink enough water. Have you ever heard someone say they get constipated despite eating a lot of bread and other high-bran sources? This is due to a lack of water consumption, a typical issue. Many of us are dehydrated all the time and are unaware of it.

It is critical to keep your body hydrated for a multitude of reasons, one of which is that water aids in the way we consume. Water is present in saliva, which contains vital enzymes that aid in correct digestion. Our saliva also moistens food, allowing us to chew it without straining our jaw. Water also plays a role in transporting food through the digestive tract. The colon is simply a minor component of the equation.

Before delving deeper into the effects of water on the colon, we must first discuss how water affects other body regions. Water is the answer if you want beautiful skin. According to studies, dehydrated people have drier and more wrinkled skin, so drink up for a more lovely outward appearance. Water also aids in our movement because our muscles would be unable to work without it. This is why athletes drink so much water. Water also helps the body combat toxins since the kidney uses water to help us eliminate toxic waste from our bodies. People who do not drink enough water are more likely to get kidney stones.

According to popular belief, the average adult needs eight glasses (64 ounces) of water daily. However, because the average adult does not weigh 120 pounds, as this statistic is predicated on, people who weigh more would require more than 64 ounces. Therefore, the amount of water you require is determined by your body weight. However, don't make the mistake of assuming that just because something is made of water, it's safe to drink. Water is used to make alcoholic beverages, for example, although, as we'll see later in this book, it's best to avoid them. Instead, drink as much pure water as possible. Tea, coffee, and other caffeinated beverages do not keep you hydrated; they dehydrate you. So, if you drink coffee in the morning, you need to drink even more water for the rest of the day.

So, what role does water play in the colon? The colon constantly absorbs water to function, and as previously indicated, fiber aids in this process. Fiber needs water to digest; drinking the appropriate amount of water will help that process. Constipation can develop when you don't drink enough water, leading to toxin buildup in the colon and other uncomfortable and life-threatening health concerns.

Intermittent Fasting

Just what is intermittent fasting? Although it's described as a diet, intermittent fasting is not an eating pattern that involves alternating between abstaining from food and caloric drinks and fasting within a specified period. To put it another way, intermittent fasting requires you to only eat at specific times.

Fasting decreases your overall calorie intake by markedly restricting or eliminating your food consumption for a determined period. Intermittent fasting is a diet system designed around the basic practice of fasting, but on a consistent and long-term basis. Intermittent fasting can be used to reach short-term weight loss goals, but it is most effective for those looking to make a lifestyle change.

Intermittent fasting offers a new approach to planning your meals while tapping into the health benefits that come along with it. There are three states of intermittent fasting; the feeding begins right when you start eating and lasts for three to five hours during digestion and absorption. This is followed by the post-absorptive state, which lasts up to 12 hours, where the body doesn't process food. Lastly, the body enters the fasting state, which begins at least nine to twelve hours after your last meal. This is the time when all manner of changes and processes take place.

Naturally, most people gravitate toward having at least three large and six small meals. Intermittent fasting offers a departure from this because you're consciously opting to go without food for a specified duration. Thus, you can either miss breakfast daily or make lunch your first meal. I'm sure you have been made to believe that breakfast is the most important meal of the day, and you should in no way skip it. Well, this eating pattern goes against such myths without putting you in harm's way.

When doing intermittent fasting, you'll need to establish your fasting and feasting windows and stick to them. This decision should be made considering your lifestyle and the ease of implementing it. For instance, if you're in a labor-intensive job, you'll do well to align your feasting window to your work hours so that you are well-energized for the day. In addition, you need to remember that unlike many diets that dictate the kinds of foods you need to eat, intermittent fasting doesn't have such restrictions. Instead, you can only eat the foods you'd normally eat, so you must be careful not to indulge in the junk.

Often described as a dieting pattern, intermittent fasting gives each person the freedom to choose how and when they want to fast to get the most out of their fasting periods. One way you have control over the program is by determining when you are going too fast. Unfortunately, people commonly misunderstand fasting because you're only doing it right if you're starving yourself. While completely avoiding food consumption is one way to fast, the more commonly practiced method where health and weight loss are concerned involves simply reducing your calorie intake during fasting times. The standard recommendation for food reduction fasting is to limit your calorie allowance to a quarter of your typical daily intake.

Not everyone who tries fasting is physically able to avoid eating entirely. Sometimes this is due to existing dietary health issues that could be negatively affected by a change in eating habits. Others, usually those new to fasting and dieting, don't have the willpower or physical stamina for this when they start. The beauty of intermittent fasting is that your body never reaches the point of starvation. You choose and adopt a fasting schedule to fit your individual needs, so there is never a period where you fast long enough that your body lacks nutrients.

At its core, intermittent fasting is something all humans already do while we sleep. So, for most, adapting to their chosen program involves prolonging this period where we aren't eating or consuming any high-calorie liquids.

Now, you may be asking yourself if it is worthwhile to make changes to when you should eat. The answer is a resounding yes. Suppose it is a great solution if you want to be lean and stay that way without having to follow crazy and difficult diet plans or focus too much on counting calories. In most cases, this eating pattern requires you to retain your calorie intake when you start.

How it works

Our bodies can handle extended periods of not eating. Human bodies have the natural ability to transition between the hungry state and the full state. When we don't eat for long, the processes going on inside our body change. When we eat, our bodies starts to digest it and store the energy received through the meal. When we are hungry, our body starts to take energy from those stored fats.

When we fast for a specific period, our blood sugar and insulin levels face a reduction in their levels. It is normal because it pushes our body to thrive from the existing resources present inside them. In addition, researchers have shown that fasting helps protect against diseases like heart disease, diabetes, cancer, and Alzheimer's disease. Therefore, you shouldn't worry that it will affect your health when in a fasted state.

Two states must be understood first to understand how intermittent fasting works. The two states are "the fed state" and "the fasted state." By understanding these states, we know how our bodies keep functioning well regardless of whether our stomachs are empty or full.

Intermittent fasting works through the combination of two phases: alternating days of eating and fasting. It is considered a more flexible approach since there are several options to choose from according to your body type, health condition, body size, nutritional needs, and weight goals. Whatever we consume is ultimately digested and metabolized into glucose, which is later used by the cells in the process of glycolysis to release energy. As it raises the blood glucose level, more insulin is produced to reduce those levels and allow the liver to initiate De Novo Lipogenesis. Lipogenesis is when the extra and unused glucose is converted into glycogen and then eventually stored as layers of fat, resulting in obesity. Intermittent fasting seems to restrict this process by deliberately causing energy deprivation, which is then met by the breakdown of the existing fat deposits.

Include Yogurt to Your Diet

Yogurt is a delectable dessert and snack that is appreciated by people all over the world. However, many people are unaware that yogurt has a high concentration of probiotics and other chemicals that aid digestion. According to scientific research, yogurt is extremely beneficial to your health, particularly your colon health. Yogurt is high in protein, vitamins, and minerals such as calcium, potassium, magnesium, and vitamins B2 and B12. A lot of contemporary studies are also focused on probiotics in yogurt. As previously established, our digestive tract contains beneficial bacteria. These beneficial bacteria help our bodies eliminate toxins and aid in food digestion. Probiotics are the bacteria that give yogurt its distinct flavor and composition in the first place, and when consumed, these beneficial bacteria settle in our intestines.

The probiotics in our digestive tract help replenish the flora that lives there. They help hasten digestion, and studies show that they improve the immune system. Some yogurt businesses claim that their product can help with irritable bowel syndrome. Yogurt does help battle gastrointestinal disorders by changing the bacteria in the intestines, so it's not simply a marketing ploy. Another marketing truth corporations love to tout is that yogurt helps women combat yeast infections. Yogurt containing active probiotics helps to adjust the pH of the blood as well as the blood sugar levels, and studies have shown that candida infections are reduced as a result. This is why many yogurt advertisements are aimed mostly at women. However, the health benefits of yogurt can be enjoyed by both men and women, young and old.

Yogurt even has ingredients that help you feel fuller after eating. In addition, people who eat yogurt before meals or as a snack eat less overall. Thus, weight loss could be another advantage of eating more yogurt.

However, not all yogurts are made equal, and many lack the living microorganisms required for a healthy colon. Always choose low-fat yogurt when shopping, as eating foods high in fat can lead to heart disease. Low-fat versions are available from well-known brands like Yoplait, Activia, and Dannon. Look carefully at the label to see if the yogurt contains live probiotic bacteria. Also, avoid eating yogurt on its own. If not previously done, combine the yogurt with fruit chunks such as fresh apples, peaches, strawberries, and blueberries. These fruits and berries are also high in fiber, which adds to their health benefits.

Consuming Colon-Harmful Foods and Substances

There are meals that you should eat and foods that you should avoid for a healthy colon. If you want a healthy colon, you should avoid eating too much fat. When you consume excess fat, your liver creates more bile acids than usual. Bile is necessary for creating feces, but too much bile in the colon can induce tumors. However, fat is not the major source of much of the colon's damage. There are a few other compounds found in foods we frequently ingest that are more harmful.

Remember how we mentioned avoiding processed and refined foods, such as those made with white flour? It turns out that eating too many refined grains can harm your gut. It's strange how washing away one small component like bran can turn a good thing like wheat into something terrible. Consuming refined grains might promote inflammation of the gut lining. These white flours are used in cakes and other sugary pastries, which can cause blood sugar levels to surge if consumed in excess. Try different grains like barley or oats if you don't enjoy whole-wheat bread. Many pasta brands contain refined grains, so avoid them or opt for a whole wheat alternative. Refined flour can also be present in the breakfast cereals we eat and provide to our children. Avoid these and instead choose cereals that contain grains, fruits, and bran. Children may not like the healthier options immediately, but you can add a favorite fruit or sweeten it slightly so they can learn to appreciate it. Make sure your rice isn't processed or refined, and pick brown rice wherever possible.

Eating a lot of red and processed meat is not a good idea. There is mounting evidence that eating too much red and processed meat increases the risk of developing colon cancer. It's scarier than it seems because it's been found that one in every five people with colon cancer ate a lot of red meat. So limit your intake of steak, beef, lamb, ham, hog, and veal. Of course, they're tasty, and it doesn't harm to indulge now and again, but control your portions for your own good. Reduce your red meat consumption to once every two weeks. Substitute vegetarian options for red meat or poultry, such as chicken and turkey. It would also help if you also considered substituting red meat with fish, as eating fish at least once a week reduces your risk of developing bowel cancer. In addition, polyunsaturated fatty acids in some fish are thought to benefit colon health. However, be aware of how you prepare and cook your fish. It has been demonstrated that cooking meats and fish at high temperatures for an extended period increases the creation of chemicals that can lead to the development of colon cancer.

Finally, stay away from alcohol. While red meat is associated with 20% of colon cancer cases, alcohol is linked to 11% of all colon cancer cases. According to research, people who drink a half pint of beer or its equivalent every day have a 20% higher risk of developing colon cancer than those who don't drink or only drink infrequently.

We hope that by devoting the previous pages to understanding how what you eat affects your colon, we have established that your diet is highly important to your colon's general health. As a result, you can now intentionally select to eat the proper types of food daily, as long as you know which other food types to avoid.

Being Active

Exercise. It is almost a cliché, but exercising can't be stressed enough because many people don't do enough of it. You can't eat exercise, but it is a natural way of ensuring that your colon stays healthy. Lack of exercise causes obesity, and studies confirm the link between obesity and cancer, especially in men. Studies show that overweight men have a 25% higher chance of developing colon cancer, while obese men have a 50% higher chance of developing colon cancer. It is not so bad for women, but exercise is equally important for men and women, and the health benefits are far-reaching.

Exercise is good for the colon as it decreases the time it takes for food to digest. This limits the amount of water taken from the feces, preventing constipation and ensuring that your poop comes out easily. In addition, when you exercise, your heart beats faster to get blood around the body since your cells need even more oxygen during this time to burn your energy stores. With the increased heart rate, richer and more oxygenated blood will be pumped into your colon, allowing your colon muscles to move even more smoothly and efficiently. This results in a more efficient digestive process, making you healthier.

The best types of exercise are those that increase your heart rate and your breathing rate. Aerobic exercises such as dancing, running, jogging, and swimming are great picks. You could also try weight training, particularly those that incorporate the core. Your regimen could include deadlifts and weighted sit-ups. For the less inclined, even simple, light exercise, such as walking, will do a lot of good for your colon and overall health. Get active, but don't overdo whatever you do, as it can hurt yourself and your colon if you exercise too much.

Given our busy lives, it is hard to find the time even to get up and walk. Instead, use your breaks to walk briskly around the office if you are at work. Go to the parking lot or a large open area and walk steadily for at least five minutes. It is even better to do this after a meal, as you will revive your colon to digest the food. But don't go too hard; you don't want to cause the blood to flow away from the colon and into the legs and arms instead.

Try to make a habit out of a daily exercise and walking regimen in the morning. Before the workday starts, mornings are often a good time to squeeze in exercise.

Eating More Fiber

One of the products that companies sell for colon cleanses is soluble fiber. Fiber is good, but what if we told you that you could get enough fiber just by eating the right foods? If you mindfully prepare and eat a balanced meal, you will get the right amount of fiber just from your diet—without spending extra money on additional fiber supplements.

Some may be wondering: what exactly is fiber, and how does it function in the body?

Think of fiber as a broom that sweeps through your colon. Fiber is the undigested part of food that helps with the formation of feces and helps promote a better-functioning colon. Yep, that is mostly it. Don't scoff, though, because what happens in your colon determines how healthy you are and how healthy you could be. Fiber comes in two forms: soluble fiber and insoluble fiber. Soluble fiber is, as you've probably guessed, fiber that dissolves in water. Bacteria ferment these fibers in the intestines and the colon into gas and other important by-products. Insoluble fiber is the form that is important for the functioning of your colon. This fiber can absorb water through the intestinal walls and bulk up your stool, making it easier to pass through the digestive system. If you don't ingest enough fiber, you are more likely to be constipated.

Soluble fibers play a huge part in processes that help keep your body healthy. For starters, these fibers reduce the absorption of sugars and normalize blood cholesterol. This is why it is bad to have high-protein meals without having the proper amount of fiber to go along with them, as you increase the chance of diseases caused by high levels of sugar, fat, and cholesterol in the body. In addition, soluble fibers bind to other substances in the body to help regulate the entrance of these same substances into the body.

Then there is insoluble fiber, which has a greater effect on the colon. These fibers also interact with other ingested substances and absorb water into fecal matter. Without it, your feces will become hard, and you will have a painful time passing your stool. The health effects of eating more fiber are enormous, and to help you understand all of them, we're going to look at the specific health benefits of fiber in your diet.

It is thought that fiber has a small role in preventing colon cancer, and current medical studies confirm this. Then there is heart disease. We have mentioned that fiber regulates the amount of cholesterol that enters the blood, and you probably know that the cholesterol buildup in the arteries causes heart disease. For many years, studies have shown that a high dietary fiber intake reduces the risk of heart disease. Scientists say that the fibers in grains are some of the most beneficial for your heart.

Another health benefit of fiber involves those diagnosed with type 2 diabetes. People with diabetes cannot process sugar like the rest of us since their insulin production is so low, leading to high blood sugar content. The fiber in the diet regulates the sugar that enters the bloodstream.

Finally, fiber helps prevent a health condition that affects most of us at least once in our lifetime: constipation. The best source of fiber for preventing constipation is wheat and oats; taking these along with a good amount of water will be very beneficial.

Fiber is found in many foods, but they tend to be the ones we like to avoid, such as our vegetables. Green vegetables such as lettuce and cabbage have high levels of fiber and other substances in them that help your digestive system. Eating them raw is best, as the cooking heat kills these important substances. However, if you don't fancy eating your vegetables raw or plain and don't like them, a more pleasant or faster way to consume them is through juicing. You get the same amount of nutrients,and if done right, vegetable juices can be delicious.

Fruits are also a good source of fiber, but unlike vegetables, the best way to consume your fruits is to eat them whole, not juice them. Fibers are mostly found in your grains and seeds, such as rice, wheat, barley, oats, etc. Unlike fruits and vegetables, the nutrients in wheat and other grains are not affected by heat. They are also okay when made into other products such as bread, cookies, and cakes. Just don't expect to get a good dietary fiber supplement from eating a black forest cake. The flour used in these cakes and most pastries is usually processed to eliminate the bran and other nutrient-containing parts of the wheat. So if you're going to eat sweet pastries and desserts, ensure that the flour is whole wheat. Another good source of fiber is rice, but make sure to choose brown rice, as white rice doesn't have the right amount of fiber either.

Legumes are the last item on our list of fiber-rich foods. Legumes include beans, peas, lentils, etc. One of the healthiest sources of fiber is green beans, as they have a high amount of fiber and low calories and carbohydrates. One of the problems with high-fiber sources is that they are rich in carbs and calories, which many people on diets aim to avoid. However, green beans are an excellent food source if you are on a low-carb diet. Other good sources of fiber include bran cereals, broccoli, spinach, cauliflower, and collard greens.

Drinking a lot of Water

Did you know that water makes up around 72% of the human body? Therefore, it makes sense to make sure you drink enough water every day. This is a more scientific breakdown of the water in your body:

- Muscles are 75% water, according to a study.
- Water makes up 82% of your blood's volume.
- Water makes up 90% of your lung tissue (no joke).
- 76% of your brain is water.
- Water accounts for 25% of your bone mass.

There are some among us who may not know the exact amount of water we should drink every day. According to a study discussed on the website of the United States National Library of Medicine, an average-sized individual (120 pounds) should consume eight to ten glasses of water daily to maintain hydration of internal organs and tissues and to wash out toxins.

Water consumption throughout the day is also highly recommended. You'll want to drink more water than usual if you have a fever, eat plenty of meat and salty cuisine, live in a dry region, or do strenuous physical activity. Take into account the following regarding your level of consumption:

Water should be used in place of sugary sodas and other unhealthy beverages whenever possible.

Herbal teas and juices with added water are fine.

Having an extra cup of water for every caffeinated or alcoholic beverage you consume is recommended.

Water can dilute digestive acids and enzymes, making food digestion more difficult; therefore, it's best to drink between meals or at least 30 minutes before and after eating.

Mealtimes are for sipping water only, and only if you really need to.

It's preferable to drink mineral water or water with a small amount of electrolyte minerals added for optimal absorption. Avoid drinking water that is too cold to avoid cramping.

One of the key benefits of drinking water is that it helps dietary fiber swell up and promotes more regular, smooth bowel movements. You don't need to be a health expert to tell you that if your bowel movements are more regular, there are fewer chances of toxins affecting your digestive system.

Is there a best time to drink water for optimum benefits? Many health experts agree that drinking water as soon as you wake up in the morning, before any food intake, can have a profoundly beneficial effect. This is a good and 100% natural way to purify your internal system. One of the most important results of practicing this method is that it helps clean your colon quickly and easily; it's free and can be done daily. As accumulated toxins are removed from your colon, your body can better absorb nutrients from your food intake.

In addition, drinking water first thing in the morning has the following benefits:

Glowing Skin - Water purges toxins from your blood, which sweeps toxins away and gives your skin that youthful glow.

Cell Renewal - New muscle and blood cell production rates are increased.

Lymph System Balance – This helps your lymph system fight infections and balance the fluids in your body.

Weight Loss - Boost your body's metabolism and remove excess waste material, allowing you to lose extra pounds.

The key to this effective method is to drink 5 to 6 glasses (1.5 liters) of water immediately after waking up. Then, avoid consuming food and other drinks (even coffee) for about an hour after drinking water. Finally, avoid alcoholic drinks before bed as they dehydrate your body.

Chia Seeds

Chia seeds are tiny, yet they are a "superfood." They are fiber powerhouses, and it is very well established in the medical community that dietary fibers have exceptional value as cleansers for our gut, including our intestines and the colon. These seeds are also very hydrating to the colon because they carry so much water that is released as they are digested. You'll see how to prepare chia seeds properly to get the most benefits in terms of both hydration and cleansing.

Chia seeds are a rich source of omega-3 fatty acids compared to other highly praised sources, such as flaxseeds. Omega-3s allow chia seeds to deliver their nutrition to the colon while reducing inflammation. Soaking chia seeds in liquids before you eat them is recommended; chia seeds develop a gelatinous coating once they are soaked, which some experts believe helps the seed move swiftly through the digestive tract.

Chia seeds are also great for reducing the risk of heart disease, strengthening bones, and providing essential nutrients like phosphorus, magnesium, manganese, copper, niacin, zinc, etc. Here are some ways you can consume chia seeds daily:

Chia seed drink: Add chia seeds to a glass of water, stir thoroughly, and once the seeds turn into gel, drink it. Get rid of the sluggishness and bloated feeling. Try adding it to coconut milk for an extra-healthy and filling drink.

Chia seed smoothie: Add chia seeds as you prepare your favorite smoothie. High in vitamin C and boasting more than 10 grams of fiber, this is a powerful antioxidant smoothie!

Sprinkle on yogurt: Sprinkle a teaspoon of chia seeds and some fruits or other healthful toppings you enjoy.

Colon Health Supplements

The majority of people in the United States take one or more dietary supplements on a daily or weekly basis. Dietary supplements nowadays might contain vitamins, minerals, herbs and botanicals, amino acids, enzymes, and a variety of additional products designed for general health and particular uses. Dietary supplements are available in several formats, including pills, capsules, powders, beverages, energy bars, gels, liquids, and gummies.

If you don't eat a diverse range of nutritious meals, several supplements may help you acquire enough critical nutrients. However, supplements cannot replace the diversity of foods essential to a healthy diet. Take dietary supplements with caution if you are pregnant or nursing, on drugs, or have a condition with which supplements may negatively interact. Most nutritional supplements have not been thoroughly evaluated for safety in pregnant women, nursing mothers, or children, and they may interact with pharmaceuticals.

When you have constipation, you may need to take supplements to help evacuate your intestines. Some people use detox with supplementation as a regular practice to clear their intestines and maintain optimum health. Let's have a look at some of the most frequent substances in colon health and detox supplements:

Aloe Vera

Aloe vera has numerous beneficial characteristics, particularly for eliminating toxins from the body. It is a thick gel with therapeutic characteristics, necessary nutrients, and herbal compounds that aid in cleaning the intestines and colon. Use aloe vera gel or juice as a colon cleanser to enhance your bowel motions and other elements of your health.

After diluting aloe juice with water, some use it as an enema to flush the colon. This can be unpleasant and difficult to accomplish on your own. Drinking aloe juice, which can contain helpful nutrients, is a better option. Most supermarkets, health food stores, and ethnic grocers stores carry bottled aloe vera, and capsules are available for various uses. It is most likely the least expensive colon-cleansing product on the list.

Cascara Sagrada

Cascara sagrada can be used alone or in combination with other herbs since it enhances the wave-like contractions of the gut muscles, which are in charge of cleaning and toning the colon. This cleaning removes toxins from the walls and provides a one-of-a-kind upkeep that prevents future buildups of these pollutants.

Although there were some questions about the safety of Cascara Sagrada, the FDA approved it as a dietary supplement. However, because of the herb's poor profitability in comparison to competing large-pharma medications, it is not yet classified as a constipation drug (which it used to be before November 2002).

Lactobacillus Acidophilus

The most common probiotic, or "good" bacteria, is Lactobacillus acidophilus (L. acidophilus). L. Acidophilus is usually found in the small intestine, which prevents potentially harmful bacteria growth.

Lactobacillus and other probiotics have been proposed to treat various ailments and disorders, including aiding digestion, curing persistent constipation, and inhibiting disease-causing bacteria.

It can also aid with lactose tolerance.

Licorice Root

This herb is extremely beneficial because it stimulates the formation of digestive juices, reduces intestinal inflammation, soothes ulcers, and activates processes that improve kidney, liver, and bladder health. It is best recognized for relieving ulcer pain and inflammation while activating the body's defensive mechanism, which keeps new ulcers from forming. To be more specific, licorice root extracts increase and reinforce the protective lining of the intestines by expanding the life span of intestinal cells and enhancing the blood supply in that region.

Licorice is especially beneficial for Lazy Bowel Syndrome (LBS), which can cause discomfort and promote illness growth in addition to clearing toxins from the intestinal tract. It has a wonderful, somewhat sweet taste and contains vitamins A, B1, B2, B5, B6, B9, and E; these nutrients are linked to improved health. The mineral benefits of licorice include calcium, iron, magnesium, phosphorus, sodium, manganese, potassium, cobalt, silicon, chrome, zinc, and selenium.

Psyllium Husk

Psyllium is a fiber-rich soluble supplement that is commonly used for colon cleansing, like the first two, and aids in the removal of bulk waste from the bowel. Various OTC (over-the-counter) supplements contain psyllium husk; it is always best to choose one that contains natural fiber extracted from psyllium plant seeds.

Consult your doctor or perform a workup to determine your appropriate dosage. Typically, 1 to 3 dosages per day are sufficient to encourage complete bowel emptying. For best results, take the recommended dosage between meals. If you take the supplement before or after meals, it may interfere with digestion.

Senna Extract

Senna is an FDA-approved laxative that is well-known for treating constipation. Professionals also extensively use it to help their patients cleanse their bowels before colonoscopies. The Senna tree contains compounds known to irritate the intestinal lining, resulting in a laxative action.

It is also used to treat IBS and as a weight-loss aid. However, the American Herbal Products Association (AHPA) has issued a warning against the long-term use of senna leaf, recommending that it be used only in emergencies. On the other hand, the fruit and fruit extract are comparably mild and deemed fully safe.

If you experience diarrhea or gastrointestinal pain, avoid using senna products. It is best to get medical advice, especially if you are pregnant or nursing a child.

What to Look for When Buying Colon Detox/Cleanse?

Dietary supplements can be complex products that are difficult to regulate. Therefore, the FDA has established good manufacturing practices (GMPs) for dietary supplements to help ensure their identity, purity, strength, and composition. These GMPs are designed to prevent the inclusion of the wrong ingredient, the addition of too much or too little of an ingredient, the possibility of contamination, and the improper packaging and labeling of a product. In addition, the FDA periodically inspects facilities that manufacture dietary supplements.

Thus, always read the labels and ensure the supplements are manufactured in GMP laboratories. Next, look for colon supplements containing Aloe Vera and Lactobacillus acidophilus (L. acidophilus), besides other common herbs that help clear toxins and excess waste.

Aloe vera has healing powers and provides essential nutrients as you clean your colon. Lactobacillus acidophilus (L. acidophilus) probiotic replaces "good bacteria," which may be lost during colon cleansing. and discourages the assembly of any other bacteria that may be harmful at the same time.

Food That Aid in Better Colon Health

Like your heart, brain, and bones, diet impacts other parts of your body, including the colon. The colon is an integral part of the human digestive system. However, conditions like inflammatory bowel disease, irritable bowel syndrome, diverticular disease, colon cancer, and ulcerative colitis can make it work improperly, leading to pain and disease.

These diseases require major lifestyle changes, medications, and sometimes even surgical procedures. Colon cancer is the third most common cancer in the United States, and the risk is higher for those over 50 years of age. Experts say that risks are also higher among obese individuals because of increased blood insulin levels. It is strongly speculated that lifestyle changes can prevent most colon cancers.

Dieticians will tell you the same thing, and we managed to get the Dos and Don'ts from an expert dietitian at the American Cancer Society.

Our bodies do not digest fiber. It remains almost the same when we pass it out, especially insoluble fiber. Soluble fiber, on the other hand, forms a gel in the stomach to slow down digestion and lower blood glucose and sugar. The role of insoluble fiber is to aid the movement of digested foods through the intestines. Regardless of their differences, they are not absorbed in our bodies, so a lack of fiber in our diet can cause constipation, high blood sugar, and diminished appetite control.

As stated on the ww.medlineplus.gov website, the daily recommended intake (DRI) for adults 19 to 50 years old is 38 grams daily for men and 25 grams daily for women. To get more variety into your diet, eat different foods, such as fruits, vegetables, and whole grains.

Examples of good fiber sources in vegetables include lettuce, raw carrots, spinach, cucumbers, and bell peppers. Tender-cooked vegetables, such as asparagus, beets, mushrooms, turnips, and pumpkin, are rich in fiber, too. You can also get more fiber by eating legumes (such as lentils, black beans, split peas, kidney beans, lima beans, and chickpeas), nuts, and seeds (such as sunflower seeds, almonds, pistachios, and pecans).

Fruits are another good source of fiber. Eat more fruits like apples, bananas, peaches, pears, tangerines, prunes, figs, and other dried fruits. For grains, go for hot cereals such as oatmeal or millet. Whole-grain bread, brown rice, and high-fiber cereals such as bran and shredded wheat are better than their highly processed counterparts.

Food to Avoid

While cleaning your colon, you must avoid processed foods, sugars, and other artificial sweeteners, as well as dairy products, which tend to produce excess mucous and can cause allergic reactions.

Most processed foods are filled with additives, loaded with excessive sugars, and stripped of nutrients. Additionally, the trans-fats present in processed food are twice as dangerous for your heart as saturated fat. So try as much as possible to avoid processed food and opt for healthier foods, like raw vegetables and fruits.

These days, processed comfort food is is widely consumed. To protect itself from processed food's acidic nature, our body coats the food with mucus. While moving through our intestines, it forms a plaque on the walls, preventing nutrients from being absorbed into our body. That is the reason why most of us start to feel hungry a short while after a meal.

Exercises and Yoga

Special exercises and yoga postures are the least you can do for a healthy colon and effective bowel movements. However, these exercises are recommended and have been proven to restore the health of your colon:

Walking, running, or jogging are some of the most basic exercises requiring no equipment or gym. However, jump rope workouts are said to increase heart rate and blood flow throughout the body. It is also claimed that the colon is automatically cleansed by jumping exercises because of the vigorous whole-body motion.

Sit-ups and crunches are effective workouts for colon health and can help with many problems, including polyps. These workouts undoubtedly tone and strengthen the abdomen and have very positive effects on the internal organs and muscles in that region. In addition, they strengthen your abdomen as a whole, helping it force the toxins out.

Jumping on a small trampoline is highly beneficial to digestive health. This is the most unconventional exercise on the list, but many people swear by it. It constantly forces the region of the abdomen to stress and release, and the tissues that hold the colon are effectively stimulated. There is honestly no motivation required to pursue this fun-filled routine, just the will to revisit childhood days. We are certain that our younger selves are alive in all of us. Some people also refer to it as "rebounding."

Exercises for a Healthy Colon

People tell me that they've completely altered their diets and now focus on having a healthy colon. However, for some reason, they continue to fall short of their health goals.

It's important to understand that diet is just one part of colon health. Colon health cannot be attained through a one-dimensional approach; you need a whole-person approach. That means making other parts of your life pro-colon, like altering your behavior, your daily routine, your sleeping patterns, and what you choose to do for exercise.

That's because exercise improves blood flow and circulation throughout the intestinal tract. It also optimizes oxygen for your colon. As a result, it enhanced the overall efficiency of the digestive system. It can even keep many colon diseases at bay. For example, regular exercise can decrease the chances of developing colon polyps (the most common colon disease) by as much as 16%.

You don't need an elaborate and complex fitness routine. Just 10 to15 minutes of exercise a day can make a world of difference. I would encourage you to bump that number up to 30 minutes daily, but one step at a time. Make time for any of these five simple exercises in your daily routine, and you should be able to notice the difference soon enough.

Walking/Jogging/Running

Walking, jogging, or running are the simplest exercises you can incorporate into your daily routine without any worries. And the best part is that they require very little to no equipment.

Walking is the lightest exercise. It is the safest exercise as well. Brisk walking or simply maintaining a quick pace will give you better results.

Jogging is more difficult than walking, but it is certainly something you can easily train your body to do. If jogging is too hard on the knees, jog on dirt or grass.

Running is probably the most effective among the above three. However, only run when you have established a good base and feel confident that you can go for a few miles without stopping.

Jumping Rope

Jumping rope is an excellent exercise that you can do anywhere. It increases heart rate and blood flow, which naturally helps overall colon health. Plus, just 10 minutes of skipping rope is the equivalent of 8 minutes of running.

Trampoline

Apart from strengthening core muscles, jumping on a trampoline also enhances peristaltic movement. Peristaltic movement is the symmetrical contraction and relaxation of muscles that lead to the movement of food inside the colon and eventually help with moving feces out of the colon.

Sit-ups and Crunches

Sit-ups and crunches are essential for strengthening your core muscles. In addition, this improves the body's ability to digest food efficiently and eliminate waste, feces, and toxins.

Though all these exercises are fairly simple, they require dedication. You can also make other changes to your routine to make it more physically challenging. For example, taking the stairs instead of an elevator, parking your car farther away from your place of work, or at the grocery store

Yoga

Yoga works in a subtle way to improve our bodies. Yoga cannot be rushed, so have patience while doing it. Yoga is also a great stress buster. The yoga poses that work best for the colon are: the hero pose, headstand, crow pose, inverted staff pose, and cobra pose.

Yoga is great for relieving stress, but every posture it has is also focused on physical improvement through stretches or balancing. Many of these are specifically great for the abdomen; these are:

- Inverted Staff Pose
- Cobra Pose
- Hero Pose
- Headstand
- Crow Pose
- Cat Pose
- Wind-Relieving Pose
- Downward-Facing Dog
- Half Sitting-Spinal Twist
- The Bow Pose
- The Garland Pose

Coffee Enema

Coffee enemas may help relieve constipation and insomnia. A coffee enema injects coffee via the anus to cleanse the rectum and large intestines. Flushing your colon with coffee stimulates the liver into producing the master detoxifying compound, glutathione S-transferase. This compound binds with all the toxins in the body and is flushed out along with the coffee.

- The amount of toxins in our bodies has increased over time, as has the need to detoxify our bodies more frequently.Coffee enemas are a strong addition to the process because:
- Studies show that it reduces toxins by up to 600%
- It cleans and heals the colon
- Increases energy levels and lifts mood
- Helps patients suffering from depression and sluggishness
- Improves digestion

Detoxifies and Repairs the Liver

You could buy an enema kit and do it yourself; however, we recommend seeking help from a professional, especially if you have never performed an enema on yourself. Always remember to use organic coffee and wait until it cools off somewhat.

How Does Exercise Affect Colon Health?

Adults should engage in at least one hour of physical activity daily for good overall health. Exercise is a boost of energy for your colon, like star power in Super Mario.

The rule of thumb is that the more active you are, the healthier your colon will be.

If you are new to exercise, start with something slow, like walking for ten minutes a day, and increase it slowly until you reach one hour.

Another activity could be punching underwater if mobility is an issue.

A good colon daily routine might look something like this:

Your day starts with waking up naturally after a restful eight-hour sleep. You first drink a lemon ginger tea with a pinch of turmeric before heading to the washroom. Next, you wait at least thirty minutes before you eat breakfast. After you return from your adventures in the restroom, you roll out your yoga mat and do a ten-minute yoga routine followed by a twenty-minute full-body routine. Finally, you drink a glass of water to stay hydrated.

Like clockwork, it's time to have a bowel movement. It's s-shaped, and no pain is present. The rumor on the street is that a bowel movement will wake you up faster than a cup of coffee. So you take a quick shower.

You start your morning mental health activity with one minute of meditation, one minute of journaling, and one minute of reading your current favorite book. You have another glass of water with vitamin D drops to stay hydrated. Getting ready for work is a breeze with your pre-selected outfit for the day. You have an egg omelet filled with veggies and a fruit smoothie for breakfast. You walk out the door, start your commute to work, and listen to a motivational music playlist. You do this to increase your energy.

You arrive 15 minutes early to work. You use this extra time to meditate for five minutes and spend the rest of the time preparing for the workday. You only work at an excellent level for your mental health, or you have an emergency protocol when your mental health is stressed. You have a great community at work, and your work-life balance is perfect for your needs and wants in life.

Lunch is your choice of meat and cooked rice with veggies and fruit. You eat meat three times a week. You are a xenophile who loves different cultures; you love exploring these cultures through cuisine.

You listen to a funk music playlist on your commute home to maintain high frequency. Then, when you arrive home, you change into your pre-selected outfit for the night and have a fruit salad while watching your shows and catching up on pop culture. Finally, you take about an hour of downtime to decompress from the workday and transition to home life.

After the well-deserved rest, you start your evening mental health activity with ten minutes of meditation, journaling, and reading your book. Then, finally, you have an early dinner: vegetable soup with a baked sweet potato for dessert.

After you finish your dinner, you give yourself one hour of me-time for your hobbies: sewing your clothes and gardening. You love how you are getting better-quality food and clothing. Because of the current climate crisis, you try to be as sustainable as possible. You are very concerned about your carbon footprint. Today you're giving yourself one hour to work on your current gardening project, growing Italian zucchini. You want to research and prepare as Italy is on your exploration on your cultural cuisine list. Tomorrow you will allocate an hour to your t-shirt sewing project; you are learning how to do a V-neckline.

You have aloe vera cubes with grapes for a snack while on your thirty-minute nature walk. You love nature; it calms you down. The sounds of the birds make you smile.

When you arrive back home, you go into your one-hour pre-sleep routine. It includes a pre-selected outfit for sleep, going to the washroom, minimal screen time, no social media, a gratitude journal, and delta binaural beats.

When you are ready, the lights are off, and with the help of blackout curtains, an eye mask, and earplugs, you fall into a beautiful eight-hour sleep.

If you want to know how to achieve this lifestyle or something close to it, from making lemon ginger tea to understanding what binaural beats are, please continue reading this book.

It's also a good idea to point out that not everything in this good daily routine needs to be done all at once. Remember to take your time and move at your own pace. Everyone will have to rewrite this story to match their exact situation. Is there anything from the story you can adopt today?

Special "Food" for More Effective Colon Cleansing

Green Foods – Love the leafy green vegetables with deep, rich color tones? They do a great deal to clean the colon and protect the digestive tract from different ailments. Part of the credit is due to the chlorophyll they contain. The high chlorophyll content in green leafy vegetables like spinach and kale promotes healthy digestion and can be eaten daily.

Fat-soluble chlorophyll adheres to the lining of the intestinal wall and inhibits bacterial growth, removes putrefied bacteria from the colon, and helps heal the mucus lining of the gastrointestinal tract. Green foods include alfalfa, wheatgrass, spirulina, green olives, celery, and sea vegetables like seaweeds. In addition to colon cleansing, chlorophyll heals damaged tissue in the digestive tract and detoxifies the liver.

Apples and Apple Cider Vinegar – "An apple a day keeps the doctor away." Do you know the apple is a powerfully cleansing fruit? Not only is it high in fiber (promotes healthy digestion), but it is rich in pectin too. Pectin helps remove built-up toxins in the colon. It also strengthens the intestinal lining at the same time.

Do you know apple cider vinegar's powerful healing and cleansing qualities were discovered in 400 B.C.? The Father of Medicine in 400 B.C. treated his patients with natural apple cider vinegar for its wonderful antibiotic and antiseptic properties that fight germs and bacteria. It is a fact that it has an alkalinizing effect on the body despite being an acidic solution.

As per some folk remedy experts, one practical method that gives such great benefit is that apple cider vinegar contains pectin, which can help soothe intestinal spasms. So now you know why many colon cleansing techniques include whole apples, apple juice, or apple cider vinegar.

Cleaning Up the Colon With Juicing

The colon, also known as the large intestine, is one of the most important organs of the digestive system. An unhealthy or dirty colon could cause various problems, such as headaches, gas, bloating, constipation, allergies, etc.

The toxins in the air, chemicals in junk food, and other such things are usually responsible for an unhealthy and dirty colon. Don't worry; good juice will clean your colon right up! Here's what you can do to make your juice cleanse more focused on the colon:

Make sure you're getting plenty of vitamin D. Your body gets this from exposure to sunlight, but it also needs vitamins K and A to absorb and process it.

Vitamins C and E Also Contribute to Colon Health

Now that you know what is good for your colon, feel free to cook unique recipes using the ingredients listed above in the fruits and vegetable section. If you are a serious juicer, you'll be able to remember what provides what in a few days. If not, you will always have this book for reference. So, I'm listing a few liver recipes of my own. Use these as a reference to create your own!

All Natural Colon Cleansing

There are plenty of all-natural, homemade options that you can use to gently and naturally cleanse your colon.

Salt Water Flush

A salt water flush must be consumed on an empty stomach first thing in the morning.

Warm about 4-8 cups of water. Add and mix 1-2 tablespoons of salt to this water. Drink the water. Try drinking it all at once. You might not feel comfortable drinking as much water for the first few weeks. Therefore, start by consuming just 2 cups. Keep increasing the quantity as you get comfortable.

Vegetable-Fruit Juice Cleanse

Pick vegetables and fruits rich in fiber and nutrients, e.g., celery, broccoli, spinach, kale, wheatgrass, apple, orange, and pear. The best combination is picking two vegetables and one fruit at a time. Puree them well in a blender until they are smooth. Please do not use a juicer, as it filters out the fiber and roughage. The water in the vegetables and fruits should be enough to give the juice a flowing consistency. You can add a little water if needed. Drink this juice every day as a meal in itself.

Green Juice

There are many green juice recipes you can make to cleanse the colon. As we said at the beginning, fiber is one of the most important components for the good functioning of the colon, and green detox drinks, if anything is left over, are fiber.

One possibility is to mix celery, parsley, lettuce, and spinach in the blender. You can add a little carrot too. However, you can vary according to what you have at home.

It must be clear that the best way to clean the colon at home is to increase the amount of fiber in the diet. Therefore, it is recommended that you review what you eat daily and increase the number of foods with fiber to cleanse the colon naturally.

For example, ensure you eat apples, raspberries, pomegranates, borage, raisins, plums, dates, whole grains, and so on.

Apart from eating more foods rich in fiber, we recommend this if you wonder how to clean the intestines and colon naturally. You need to do a deep cleaning; for example, in cases of severe constipation or toxin retention, it will be good to include in your diet some plants with high amounts of fiber.

Chapter 6: Probiotics

Probiotics consist of bacteria already present in the gut or added to a product during the fermentation process (like yogurt). Probiotics are good for you, and they include bacteria like Bifidobacterium and Lactobacillus. Live microorganisms that provide health benefits when consumed enough are a reliable definition of probiotics. Probiotics, often good or helpful bacteria, can be found in yogurt, suppositories, and nutritional supplements. Depending on the product, you may find that probiotics include a single strain of bacteria or a combination of bacteria and fungi. Since probiotics have not yet been approved for their health claims, they can only be sold as dietary supplements.

Clinical studies for probiotics have become increasingly intriguing in recent years as scientists have learned more about the human microbiome. Probiotics have been shown to have curative and preventative effects on children and adults with diarrhea and irritable bowel syndrome. In addition, probiotics have shown encouraging effects, including the prevention and reduction of necrotizing enterocolitis, a severe intestinal illness in preterm neonates. In the future, probiotics may be used to manage obesity, lower cholesterol, and control symptoms of irritable bowel syndrome. Probiotics have many possible impacts, including synthesizing antimicrobial substances and suppressing pathogenic bacteria through increased competition for nutrients and prebiotics.

Surprisingly, probiotics do not necessarily need to survive to have an effect; they can sometimes affect the behavior of the bacteria in your gut even if they do not survive. As for the major issue with probiotics, there's a lot more talk about them than proof that they work.

When was the last time you shopped for probiotics? A growing trend in grocery stores is to devote a whole aisle to probiotics and other bacteria that are said to be good for your digestive system. But at this time, there is still a shortage of hard evidence to back up these assertions. While some of the ideas that have led to the isolation of certain microorganisms are valid, the majority have not been demonstrated to be effective under these circumstances. Furthermore, given that these preparations are imported, then sit on the shelf in the store, and we know that these microorganisms require extremely precise circumstances, it is still questionable if they contain any living organisms.

The main issue, though, is that many believe any probiotic will do the trick, which is not a belief we would have for any other product. For example, let's say you were feeling under the weather, and you mentioned to a friend that you had heard of a medicine that would help and decided to try it. You can count on them to scrutinize your every move, wondering which drugs you used and why you chose them. They could also inquire about the drug's source and whether or not you have any medical evidence that it is helpful for your condition.

Though this is just one case, it illustrates how valuable scientific inquiry can be in medicine. Therefore, it is beneficial to inquire with your pharmacist about a probiotic that has undergo nerigorous scientific testing. If none of these options work, consuming live yogurt is safe and has helped many people. However, the clinical evidence reveals that even different types of live yogurt vary considerably in how much they can assist.

Benefits of Probiotics

Bacteria are everywhere, from the air we breathe to the water we drink to the food we eat. They are on your clothes and skin. Most bacteria are good and beneficial for our health. Bacteria are microbial scavengers;they eat what is not alive. They recycle the basic building blocks of life to be used again to feed the creation of new life.

Imagine a world without bacteria. Nothing would decompose. We would have the dead carcasses of dinosaurs from 50 million years ago here. Dead trees and plants would not decompose without bacteria. The oceans would be filled with dead fish. Without bacteria, the whole world would have died a long time ago. In fact, without bacteria to recycle what dies, it would not even be possible for human beings to exist on planet Earth today.

Good bacteria are on our skin, mouth, and intestines, which are essential for a normal immune system. Antibiotic soaps destroy friendly flora on our skin and make us more vulnerable to harmful bacteria. In addition, our skin is the largest organ for eliminating waste and toxic byproducts of cellular metabolism.

Activated white blood cells of our immune system reside in the lymph nodes of our intestines. Specific types of white blood cells, like macrophages, monitor digestion's byproducts and seek to block foreign proteins from entering the blood supply. The health of the digestive system (from the mouth to the colon) is the foundation for a balanced immune system for disease prevention.

Health stresses occur when undigested proteins or partially digested proteins are absorbed into the blood supply — a condition known as leaky gut syndrome exists. This causes inflammatory immune reactions that create food sensitivities and food allergies to develop. An abundance of friendly flora in the gut creates an inner garden that crowds out the weeds — the unfriendly flora, including yeast overgrowth, molds, parasites, etc.—that cause adverse health effects.

Natural wild strains of intestinal flora come from many sources, including raw mother's milk, kefir, yogurt, cheese, sauerkraut, and cultured vegetables. In addition, small amounts exist naturally on the surface of most fruits and vegetables.

Foods Rich In Probiotics

A lot of people take probiotic supplements. While nutritional supplements may deliver some benefits, the dosage and efficacy of probiotics in supplements are not guaranteed. For example, a study on 55 different brands of probiotic supplements discovered that only 13% delivered the number of probiotics listed on the packaging. Moreover, it is not always guaranteed that the preservation process will not damage the probiotics contained in the supplements. Probiotics are particularly more delicate than most other nutrients because they are 'alive,' i.e., 'living microorganisms.' Therefore, they are best obtained through food.

Most foods containing probiotics are 'cultures.' These foods are derived from a primary food source and fermented to get the benefit of probiotics from the end product. Fermenting food is not a modern technique. In ancient times, foods were fermented to preserve them or derive a new food or condiment from them.

Fermentation breaks down food molecules into a more basic form: bacteria convert carbohydrates to lactic acid, and yeast turns sugar into alcohol. Also, some people erroneously believe that probiotics are only available through dairy products, which is untrue. There are non-dairy sources of probiotics, and these are great for lactose-intolerant people.

Any food source we decide to use to increase our dose of probiotics has to be natural or organic. Many food preservation processes destroy probiotics. Avoid processed foods, particularly those that have been pasteurized. They will not deliver an adequate quantity or quality of probiotics. It is not hard to find at least one food that can supply your body with a healthy dose of probiotics, no matter what part of the planet you live on. Let'slook at some of the foods that are rich in probiotics.

<u>Aged Cheese</u>

Cheese has recently received a lot of bad press, mainly for having high cholesterol and encouraging obesity. However, we are prone to forget that certain people, such as the French, eat much more cheese than the rest of us, have remained leaner, and have had fewer incidences of cardiovascular disease than Americans.

One or two ounces of cheese per day is an excellent starting point. Choosing naturally fermented cheese over products injected with germs by the producer is recommended. Cheese prepared from raw, unpasteurized goat or cow milk and aged cheese is the finest source of probiotics. That being said, cheese labeled 'organic,' 'made from raw milk,' or 'probiotic' is always your best bet.

Lactic acid bacteria, which are helpful to our health, are abundant in naturally fermented cheese. Cheese is essentially fermented milk curds, and the starter germs used, the procedure, and the amount of fermentation time vary depending on the type of cheese. As a result, different species of lactic acid bacteria will be found in different types of cheese.

Cheese's low acidity and high fat content make it an ideal medium for good bacteria to flourish and even be carried throughout the digestive system without being destroyed.

The general guideline for cheese is that any form of cheese can be high in probiotics as long as it is not heated or pasteurized after it is manufactured. However, the cheese will only provide good probiotics to the body if it is not cooked before consumption.

Chocolate, Dark

Dark chocolate that is organic, raw, and unprocessed offers numerous health benefits and is even considered a health food. Cocoa was even referred to as the "food of the gods" by the Mayans. The ancient Aztecs mashed cocoa seeds with spices to make a drink they thought would promote good health, and they were correct.

Dark chocolate is frequently considered to include probiotics, but it is a wonderful natural 'protector' of probiotics. Thus, it works well when mixed with probiotic foods like yogurt to retain the good bacteria when we eat them.

Dark chocolate is made from cocoa powder containing two flavonol molecules called catechin and epicatechin. It also has a small amount of fermented dietary fiber. Beneficial gut bacteria can break down large polyphenolic polymers into smaller anti-inflammatory compounds that are easily absorbed by the body.

Probiotics can be found in a variety of foods. The issue is that our stomach acids typically destroy these creatures before they reach the big intestine. Dark chocolate has an advantage over some of these probiotic food sources in that it can transfer probiotics directly to the large intestine without being damaged by the acidity of stomach secretions. Dark chocolate is a natural stomach acid protector that protects against biosalts and damaging probiotics.

You can't go wrong with adding dark chocolate to your diet based on the findings of a study into dark chocolate. To reap the most nutritional benefits, consume dark chocolate with at least 70% cocoa content and no more than 3 ounces (85 grams) per day. [22] Finally, because most of us have grown accustomed to the flavor of regular chocolate, it may take some time for our taste receptors to adjust to dark chocolate. First, take little bites at a time, then gradually increase your intake.

Green Pickles

The ordinary pickle is a strong source of probiotics, despite being widely available and widely assumed. Pickles are simple to prepare if you don't want to buy commercially available ones, and they taste fantastic.

Pickles that don't include vinegar and are processed without heat are your best bet for a probiotic boost. Vinegar pickling, which involves soaking green vegetables in vinegar/acetic acid, dramatically reduces the formation of harmful microorganisms and yeast in the pickles.

Unfortunately, a large majority of commercially sold pickles are made with vinegar because doing so significantly increases the shelf life of the pickle. The exceptions include half-sour pickles, typically produced in vinegar-free brine and stored chilled in health food stores. As a result, they are frequently more expensive than if they were created at home.

The best pickles are created from fermented water, spices, and brine. When you combine green veggies in a jar in your kitchen with salt, water, and seasonings, the vegetables produce lactic acid, which preserves them. These acids are produced naturally as a byproduct of fermentation. This procedure, known as 'Lacto-fermentation,' is the conventional manner of creating pickles without vinegar. The sugars in brine-soaked greens attract to the surface and mix with lactic acid bacteria to form lactic acid, which gives the food its distinct flavor and keeps it edible for a longer period. Pickles, like most fermented foods, are high in probiotics.

Shorter fermentation times of a few weeks usually result in green pickles that are half sour, but longer fermentation periods result in lighter-colored pickles that are sourer.

Pickles can be consumed as a snack on their own or in sandwiches, hamburgers, hotdogs, and salads. And because pickles may be eaten cold, you are guaranteed to consume the probiotics they contain.

Kefir

Kefir (sometimes spelled kefir or kephir) is gaining popularity among health food lovers worldwide and for a good cause. It is a fermented drink produced by combining kefir grains with goat or cow milk and fermenting it for 24 to 48 hours. The lactic bacteria in the kefir seeds convert the lactose in the milk into lactic acid during this period. Then, the milk is drained, and the gel-like kefir grains (which resemble cauliflower) can be reused to ferment milk into kefir. The strained milk tastes similar to sour yogurt but is thinner in consistency.

The origins of kefir grains have remained a mystery, with various theories or anecdotes attempting to explain how they came to be. They were referred to as "food from the gods" in ancient times. According to one explanation, it came from sheep's mouths or intestinal germs. Another story is that shepherds carrying milk in leather and wineskin pouches discovered that it was periodically fermented, producing an effervescent drink. Another legend from the Caucasian mountains is that it was a gift from the Islamic prophet Mohammed, who instructed his followers how to use it and forbade them from exposing the secret of its preparation to anybody; hence, they are known as 'grains of the prophet.' The enigma surrounding how kefir has been manufactured is a blessing in disguise because scientists have yet to unravel it, making it one of the world's most unadulterated, authentic meals.

Kefir is not only abundant in nutrients, but it is also high in probiotics. Kefir grains contain 30 - 35 different strains of yeast and bacteria, making them more probiotic-rich than yogurt. Lactobacillus kefir is a probiotic found exclusively in kefir.

One significant advantage of kefir is that it is well-accepted by lactose-intolerant people. Aside from that, kefir is extremely flexible. Nondairy liquids like fruit juice or coconut water can also make it. Making your own kefir is a terrific idea. It is quite simple to make. Commercially accessible kefir is typically not fermented for an extended period, and pasteurization drastically reduces the probiotics in the drink. [9] When producing kefir, use milk from grass-fed cows or goats to get the most probiotics into the drink.

Some users also recommend that kefir be introduced gradually into your diet, with intake gradually increasing over time. Ingesting excessive amounts right away may result in unfavorable effects.

Kombucha

This is a probiotic-rich Asian fermented tea that has been consumed for centuries. There are numerous testimonials to its effectiveness. It is said to improve immunity, aid in weight loss, boost metabolism, promote detoxification, and relieve joint pain.

Health enthusiasts cannot avoid the sugar in kombucha because it is what the SCOBY technically 'eats' to break down and produce probiotics. Another new trend is to use decaffeinated tea instead of regular black tea to reduce the caffeine content of kombucha.

One thing to keep in mind about kombucha is that it may make you feel worse before it makes you feel better. Another way to look at it is that the bad bacteria will reject any good bacteria introduced to your body. Kombucha does not agree with everyone at first and may even worsen symptoms in some diseases before providing relief. Starting with tiny amounts can assist in alleviating this condition.

Pregnant women, children aged 10 and under, and people taking blood thinners are also advised not to consume kombucha. It is recommended to consume 4 to 8 ounces per day.

Miso

Miso has been a staple for over 2,500 years, from ancient China through Japan and currently. It is a savory, flavor-packed paste that may be used as a soup condiment. It is thought to have anti-aging properties and can negate the effects of smoking, radiation, and air pollution in the human body.

Miso is a paste or culture that is created by blending cooked, powdered soybeans, koji, salt, and water into a paste that is then formed into balls and fermented in a jar for up to six months to two or three years. The longer miso is fermented, the greater the final product's quality, as well as its richer, more nuanced flavor. The Japanese have honed their art in the production of miso.

Miso paste is an extremely versatile spice. Aside from soups, it can be used in fish or meat sauces and homemade salad dressings. When using miso, remember that it is typically heavy in salt. Our daily sodium allowance is 2,400 milligrams, and a teaspoon of miso contains around 250 grams of salt. You would probably need to eliminate or reduce the amount of salt in your recipe or use miso sparingly. Miso should be avoided by anyone who is allergic to soy.

Miso's fermentation process, combined with the infusion of koji, guarantees that it contains a sufficient amount of probiotics. Miso should be used after any cooking process so that the heat does not kill the beneficial microorganisms it contains. Unpasteurized miso is preferable, and storing it in an airtight container in the fridge is the best method to keep it fresh.

Olives

Olives are delicious appetizers and one of the most nutrient-dense fruits on the planet. Their high monounsaturated fat content benefits the brain, heart, and waistline. They are also high in antioxidants, specifically biophenols, which help keep harmful cholesterol from clogging the arteries. The nutritional value of olives increases over time. Because they are fermented, olives are high in lactobacillus, or gut-friendly bacteria. [30] Eating them is a great way to reap the benefits of these beneficial microorganisms. Remember that olives are normally soaked in brine, so reducing the salt in any cuisine they present is a good way to minimize excessive salt consumption.

Sauerkraut

Some people have difficulty digesting cabbage. Therefore, sauerkraut is an excellent substitute. Sauerkraut is also an excellent source of probiotics for people who are lactose intolerant and need to supplement their diet with probiotics. Again, like most other probiotic food sources, commercially marketed sauerkraut is frequently pasteurized, so it has no microbial nutrients. The best sauerkraut is homemade.

Sauerkraut translates to "sour cabbage" in German. It is a type of 'pickled cabbage' created by chopping, crushing, and pressing or squeezing the cabbage with salt [14] to remove its water or juice, then preserving it in a jar with the juice drained for around twelve days to three months. When the cabbage is ready to eat, it turns from green to pale yellow.

Sauerkraut can be eaten hot or cold, but if you want to obtain the probiotics from it, eat it cold because heat kills the probiotic content. Sauerkraut can be eaten cold in a variety of ways. Include it as a stuffing in hot dogs or sandwiches, add it to cold salads, potato dishes, eggs, fish, or meat, or serve it as a condiment to the main course. Some folks include sauerkraut in their vegetable smoothie. Sauerkraut juice is even sold as a digestive tonic on its own.

Sauerkraut is a surprisingly rich probiotic source, providing a significant nutritional benefit. Sauerkraut ranks first on the list of probiotic-rich foods. It is reported to have more probiotics per gram than any dairy product or over-the-counter supplement. Studies have been undertaken to back up this startling conclusion regarding sauerkraut.

Compared to yogurt, which contains roughly 100 million probiotics per 100 grams, sauerkraut has a whopping 10 trillion grams of probiotics per 100 grams!

Sauerkraut, in addition to probiotics, contains a variety of additional nutrients, including vitamin A and up to 200 times more vitamin C than a head of cabbage. You have nothing to lose by eating this delicious meal.

They have been farmed for decades as food and are sometimes available in powder form.

Microalgae is consumed by millions of Asians, Olympic competitors, and even NASA astronauts for the excellent nutrients it provides. Spirulina has approximately 65% protein, and chlorella contains approximately 45% protein. They also provide other nutrients, such as carbs, fiber, vitamins, and minerals, when combined.

Spirulina is a safe nutrient source that has been utilized for many years. It is reported to have detoxifying effects in addition to being nourishing. Chlorella resembles spirulina in appearance and can help eliminate heavy metals from the body and improve liver health. [19] The high chlorophyll content aids digestion and contains high levels of protein, antioxidants, and easily absorbed vitamins. They are also high in energy and boost your vigor when taken.

In recent years, the practice of incorporating spirulina and chlorella into fermented milk products such as yogurt to boost probiotic activity has grown in popularity. Microalgae like these can improve the viability of probiotics in fermented dairy products like yogurt.

According to one study, the addition of spirulina and chlorella to fermented milk not only boosted the viability of probiotics in the product but also the functional characteristics of the probiotic. (2013) (Beheshtipour, Mortazavian, Mohammadi, Sohrabvandi, and Khosravi-Darani) This is because these two microalgae include a wide spectrum of nutrients and nutraceuticals; consequently, they are "functional foods." Functional foods are simply foods that have health-promoting ingredients.

Microalgae are a dense source of powerful nourishment that may be incorporated into your diet in various ways. It is claimed that the number of microalgae contained in a little tablet-size supplement (which may be similar to half a teaspoon of powdered algae) can provide give the same amount of nourishment as eating salads all day long. It can be mixed into smoothies, shakes, yogurts, milk, peanut butter, sandwiches, or chewed and eaten with water.

Tempeh

Tempeh is produced from whole soya beans that have had their husks removed before being partially boiled, mashed, and fermented with mold. The mold breaks down the soy meal and bonds its molecules into a cake-like structure during fermentation. Vegans and vegetarians frequently utilize tempeh as a substitute for beef, bacon, or tofu.

It is thought to have originated in Indonesia several centuries ago. It is now eaten all over the world. Tempeh, made solely from soya beans, is popular in Indonesia. In other parts of the world, soya bean for tempeh are sometimes combined with grains such as millet and barley.

The fermentation process that tempeh goes through makes it easier to digest and absorb. Some say it has a savory and nutty flavor as sweet and earthy.

Tempeh can be served in a variety of ways. It can be cooked in various ways, including boiling, frying, and grilling. It is available in practically every market and village in Indonesia. It can be cooked and eaten at home in rice or soups and is also available on the menus of the world's greatest fine dining establishments. It can also be grilled, stir-fried, or used as a sandwich filler substitute.

Tempeh patties can be used in place of beef in hamburgers. It's also in an Asian sauce. Kimchi is occasionally made using tempeh.

This Asian fermented cabbage is often given as an addition to many meals, such as rice, soup, dumplings, and rolls, particularly in Korea. It can best be described as a hotter and slightly sour-tasting variety of sauerkraut.

Lacto-fermentation occurs during this time. Lactobacillus bacteria convert the sugars in cabbage to lactic acid, giving the cabbage a new, sour flavor. When fermented, kimchi is best stored in the refrigerator.

Kimchi is simple to make and comes in a variety of flavors. Some individuals flavor their kimchi with additional ingredients like sugar, carrots, garlic, ginger, kelp powder, seafood taste, and so on. Some people want it hot, while others prefer it mild; therefore, when making your kimchi, you may control the heat by reducing or increasing the amount of gochugaru you use.

It is recommended that small amounts of kimchi be ingested at a time. People with high blood pressure should consume significantly less kimchi than the average person due to its high salt content.

Yogurt Live Cultured

Yogurt is the first meal that comes to mind when seeking a high-probiotic source. Unfortunately, the issue with yogurt is that most commercially available yogurt is pasteurized, loaded with sugar and additives, and contains no probiotics.

Even when it comes to more organic products and unsweetened varieties like Greek yogurt, not all brands are created equal. Some higher-quality brands may even deliver fewer probiotics than lower-quality brands.

Natural, organic, unprocessed yogurt is the best source of probiotics. The probiotic activity orcontent in refined, sweetened, and fancy packaged yogurts is negligible. Homemade, unprocessed yogurt contains a high concentration of probiotics. Yogurt made from goat milk is claimed to have a high probiotic content.

Several studies have been undertaken, and it has been discovered that yogurt consumption is advantageous to digestive health (Irritable Bowel Syndrome (IBS) and diarrhea), upper respiratory infections, and even brain health. The main stipulation is that regular ingestion, rather than infrequent usage, is essential before any substantial improvements may be observed.

In addition to probiotics, yogurt contains animal protein and other essential nutrients, such as vitamins and minerals. Lactose-intolerant people can also drink yogurt.

Yogurt is fantastic since it can be eaten on its own or mixed with other delights, desserts, and smoothies. However, the probiotic component is destroyed if yogurt is heated before usage. Therefore, it tastes the finest chilled or, at most, at room temperature.

Wheat Grasses

Most sprouted seeds and grains are nutritionally dense. Wheatgrass is made from wheat seeds and is rich in chlorophyll and fiber. The combination of chlorophyll and fiber is beneficial to colon health and necessary for probiotics to grow and keep us healthy. Wheatgrass can be juiced or dried and made into a powder, then added to shakes or smoothies for optimal nourishment.

Buttermilk

Buttermilk is a byproduct of the buttermaking process. Milk divides into two parts when churned: butter and whey. The whey is commonly referred to as buttermilk. When traditionally manufactured, whey contains naturally existing lactic acid bacteria that aid in the fermentation of the milk before it is churned. As a result, it has a strong acidic flavor that works well in various foods, particularly pancakes, pastries, and pudding, and as an alternative in yogurt dishes. To get the most out of the healthful bacteria it contains, it should be consumed cold or in cold meals such as salads, desserts, or as a side dish to the main course. Store-bought buttermilk is usually pasteurized and made from cultured skim milk Therefore, buying traditional buttermilk from health food stores is ideal; make sure it's organic and says "live culture" on the label.

Bread with Sourdough

This is a sort of bread that has been created from the start and has been fermented for at least one day or more before being kneaded with other ingredients to make bread. The fermentation procedure yields a starter that is abundant in helpful microorganisms. As a result, many people assume that sourdough bread contains a high amount of probiotics. The difficulty with this assumption is that the heat required to bake bread would kill most microorganisms. More research is needed to back up the claims of probiotics in sourdough bread.

Beer

Commercially accessible beers are not always probiotic since, despite being generated through a fermentation process, the yeasts and live bacteria in them are usually killed near the conclusion of the production process when they are pasteurized. Beer from living cultures is usually darker, unfiltered, unpasteurized, less common, and more expensive, but it must be taken in moderation to reap any health advantages. They often have a greater alcoholic content [31] and, like wine, can be matured due to their live cultures. The flavor improves as it ages, and the alcohol content rises.

Natto

This is a stringy, fermented soya bean Japanese dish with a characteristically pungent aroma and flavor. It is high in probiotics, especially Bacillus subtilis, formerly known as Bacillus natto. Natto and rice are popular breakfast dishes in Japan, but they are also found in sushi, salads, and even burritos. It is high in vitamin K and a good source of plant protein. Natto is sometimes combined with a sweet sauce that is high in fructose. The healthier way to eat natto is to skip the sauce and instead use soy sauce.

Chapter 7: Is it Really Important to Do a Colon Clean Cleanse?

Toxins and waste materials tend to accumulate in the colon when its function is impaired. It's more likely that your body will absorb substances if they take longer to reach their destination. Whenever this occurs, it's possible to develop or suffer from a wide range of illnesses.

Many different kinds of potentially infectious microbes are encountered by the colon on a daily basis. The figures may approach the billions. There are both hazardous and helpful types of bacteria. In a well-functioning gut, beneficial bacteria would outnumber pathogenic ones. If not, harmful bacteria could proliferate and destroy the beneficial microbes in the body.

When harmful bacteria infiltrate the colon, normal bowel function may be disrupted. When bacteria take over, a wide range of abnormalities can manifest in the body. Constipation, diarrhea, Crohn's disease, colitis, and irritable bowel syndrome are all examples.

Colon cleansing is one of the most efficient methods for maintaining a healthy digestive system and overall health. It's as simple as eating more fiber-rich meals, drinking enough water, and getting some exercise on a regular basis. Including the proper amounts of vitamins and minerals in your diet is also beneficial.

What Options Exist For Colon Detoxification At Home?

If you're considering colon cleansing at home, you're not alone. Before you, millions of others have cleansed their colons. In addition, colon cleansing has received much interest in recent years. Continue reading to learn more about colon cleansing at home. The purported benefits of colon cleansing include:

Colon cleansing can help cleanse the body of accumulated toxins in the digestive tract and colon. Many individuals have claimed favorable outcomes from at-home colon cleansing. People who have tried colon cleansing solutions say they no longer get headaches.

Many individuals who have attempted colon cleansing at home report feeling significantly more energized. They no longer feel exhausted. Others have stated that after cleaning their colons, their constipation was alleviated. Many individuals who have undergone a colon cleanse report feeling better after the procedure.

Home colon cleansing was not always available. Therefore, colonic hydrotherapy was the only method available to cleanse the colon. This colon cleansing method involves sending around 20 gallons of water through a tube placed in the colon.

All of this is performed by a professional technician. The waste buildup is eliminated by the pressured water delivered through the tube and into the colonThis technique is still in use today.

You might not want someone, especially a stranger, to pump water into your intestines. Fortunately, there is a method for getting a clean colon without using pressurized water or a stranger. There are two alternative natural methods for cleansing the colon at home.

How to Make a Homemade Colon Cleansing System to Eliminate Toxins?

The accumulation of toxins in the colon causes different diseases. Consequently, colon cleansing is important. A clean colon indicates good general health and a healthy digestive tract. There are several different ways to cleanse your colon. You can purchase a colon cleansing kit consisting of powders and tablets or make one yourself.

However, most colon cleansing regimens leave you malnourished. Therefore, you must also take certain vitamins to maintain general health while on a colon cleansing plan. It is recommended that you add acidophilus (a probiotic) to the DIY colon cleanse to restore the digestive system's beneficial flora. Egg yolks and yeast flakes are excellent alternatives to multivitamins. A vitamin C pill reduces negative effects such as brain fog and fatigue.

Juice cleanses are also an efficient method for eliminating toxins from the intestines. Be sure to use fresh vegetables and fruits instead of store-bought artificial juices. They must be made from scratch. Juice cleanses also require enormous amounts of water, which assist in flushing out accumulated toxins.

Psyllium powder and bentonite clay (P&B) shakes are one of the most popular homemade colon cleanses. Clay serves as a binder, and psyllium offers the fiber. Together, these potent substances eliminate parasites and harmful waste from your intestines.

After obtaining your P&B shake, you may consume one shake every day for one week. Then, increase the amount gradually until you can consume three to five P&B shakes every day. However, patience is essential. A P&B colon cleanse produces visible results within a few months.

It is recommended that the P&B shake be had at least one hour before a meal on an empty stomach. Add probiotics to your colon cleansing plan. The body requires beneficial bacteria, but the P&B shakes eliminate all germs, including the good ones. Dietary adjustments must also be considered when performing colon cleansing. Consume a diet rich in fruits and vegetables and low in refined grains and sugar.

A colon can assist with persistent acne, glycemic index (GI) issues, weight issues, and energy levels. Both decent homemade colon cleanses and commercial colon cleansing kits are quite helpful in addressing different bodily issues. However, commitment is required when beginning a colon cleansing regimen. When preparing a DIY colon cleanse, even more commitment is required.

Herbs cleansing the colon:

Nature has gratefully provided us with several plants that can aid colon cleansing. Among these plants are:

- Psyllium hulls,
- Grapefruit pectin,
- Licorice root,
- Flax seeds and
- Rhubarb root.

There are many more than those listed above. Using the herbs mentioned above can cause stomach pain in certain individuals. If you intend to use the above herbs to cleanse your colon at home, it is highly recommended that you stay hydrated by drinking lots of water. In addition, it would be best to refrain from eating for 24 to 48 hours while taking the colon-cleansing herbs.

Ready-made Products for Colon Cleansing:

Although the herbs mentioned above will help you cleanse your colon at home, it might be difficult to determine the ideal combination and dosage. Also, it is difficult to maintain a program of taking the necessary herbs for a good colon cleansing in today's fast-paced environment.

To obtain a clean colon, will you be compelled to endure pressured water from a stranger? No, there is a simpler, more economical alternative; you can use a ready-made, all-natural colon cleansing product.

For most people, colon cleansing at home with a ready-made solution is the best option. It is considerably more convenient to purchase a premade item. These products often comprise the herbs mentioned above in sufficient quantities to cleanse the colon and digestive tract.

Advantages of Colon Cleansing

Preparing for surgery involving the colon, such as a colonoscopy, often necessitates a colon cleanse.

Every day, the body gets rid of a lot of waste products. Some toxins, however, are tenacious, making disposal a major hassle. Colon cleansing is extremely effective for these poisons.

As a result of their low cost and relative safety, natural or herbal cleansers are widely used by those interested in colon cleansing.

Yet another miraculous substance is psyllium husk, a byproduct of the plant plat. Most commercially available dietary supplements to cleanse the colon contain this husk.

Improved immunity is another benefit, as is increased energy afterward.

Disadvantages

There hasn't been enough systematic study of the advantages and disadvantages of scientists. However, there are some drawbacks to a colon cleanse, according to research.

The risk of the body entering a state of extreme dehydration increases when the colon is cleansed. A severe water and mineral imbalance can devastate one's health.

Colon cleansing has many negative side effects, including dehydration, cramping, dizziness, vomiting, nausea, bowel perforation, and allergic reactions.

Products claiming to clean out the colon typically tout themselves as risk-free. Neither their safety nor their efficacy have been established through medical testing, so they are not subject to any laws governing the sale of consumer goods. Users take full responsibility for any consequences resulting from their reliance on them.

Numerous people advertise themselves as colon cleansing specialists, but none have official certification or training.

Theoretically, a colon cleanse sounds great, but we can't be sure until more research is done. The lack of conclusive evidence makes it possible that colon cleansing does more harm than good.

This is why you should only do a colon cleanse if your doctor recommends it. In addition, a cleanse should only be performed by a qualified professional. If you're set on getting "cleaned up," the best place to start is by eating and living healthily to purge your colon. Increase your intake of water and fiber, exercise regularly, and make time for meditation.

The Benefits Of Colon Cleansing To Your Overall Health.

Colon cleansing offers significant health benefits, no doubt. However, in reality, many cleaning health benefits have been clinically demonstrated. In addition, people increasingly recognize the benefits of a healthy colon, so they opt for cleansing procedures.

Constipation.

Constipation is among the most common issues associated with an unhealthy colon. In reality, many constipation sufferers are unaware of their condition. Over 400 million dollars are spent yearly on laxatives; this is only for the United States.

One of the primary advantages of cleansing is that it improves the gastrointestinal system. Thus, it assists in treating and preventing constipation. In addition, this procedure assists in the removal of solidified feces from the large intestine, allowing for the efficient evacuation of waste. Constipation is, in reality, one of the primary causes of a sick colon. Therefore, regular colon cleansing improves the health of the colon and your general health.

Diarrhea.

Also, cleansing is a good treatment for diarrhea. Diarrhea is your body's reaction to the accumulated poisons. First, the body is dehydrated by rushing water into the colon to clear waste. If your colon is healthy, your body will not need to flush out toxins. Therefore, you would not experience diarrhea.

Weight Loss.

Although colon cleansing is not directly linked to weight loss, it does result in weight loss. This is because it assists in eliminating all collected feces, hence assisting in weight loss. A healthy individual is estimated to carry between 5 and 20 pounds of feces in their colon.

Colon Carcinoma.

Also, it lessens your risk of developing colon and rectal cancer. Colon cleansing helps maintain a healthy and smooth colon. Those with a history of colon or rectal cancer in their family should undergo frequent colon cleansing.

In addition to these well-known health benefits of colon cleansing, there are other lesser-known health benefits linked with colon cleansing.

Everyone wants clean, healthy skin, but women especially. Colon cleansing improves the texture and feel of our skin significantly. In addition, it helps eliminate skin issues such as acne.

Colon cleansing is beneficial to our overall health. It improves the performance of all organs by removing pollutants from our bodies. When toxins are removed from the body, the metabolic and endocrine systems improve significantly. After undergoing a colon cleansing, your energy level will increase dramatically. Moreover, you feel more energized.

In addition, it improves the absorption of nutrients from the food you eat. If you suffer from a nutritional deficiency, colon cleansing will improve your body's ability to absorb vitamins, minerals, proteins, lipids, and carbs.

Your concentration will also increase as a result of the cleansing.

Also, cleansing eliminates parasites from the body. These parasites create severe health problems if permitted to persist in the body for an extended period. Therefore, it is beyond question that colon cleansing improves our overall health. It enables us to live a disease-free and healthy life.

Do Colon Cleansing Weight Loss Programs Work?

Colon cleansing weight loss treatments are growing in popularity. Many individuals are becoming aware of how many pollutants they are exposed to daily. Many factors negatively impact our health and quality of life.

Many diseases are on the rise, and new diseases are identified daily. Therefore, it is time to examine how we may minimize our exposure and control the aspects of our lives that will benefit us. For example, consider the American diet, which comprises refined and processed foods that might be filled with chemicals and preservatives.

We consume fatty and sugary fast foods and fried foods. Toxins are ubiquitous. Our produce is farmed using chemicals and pesticides. Our meat contains antibiotics and hormones. Our air and water are polluted, and the list continues.

Our bodies were meant to detoxify and cleanse, yet each individual has a different toxic threshold based on their circumstances. For example, when we regularly consume foods lacking in nutrients and fiber, the food can pass through the body without being fully digested and removed.

When food is not expelled from the body promptly, it sits in the gut for too long, allowing it to rot and ferment. The longer this muck remains in the colon, the more it is reabsorbed by the blood. Therefore, using a colon cleanse for weight reduction is an excellent option.

The benefits are that it is easy and inexpensive, and you will undoubtedly lose weight.

The disadvantages are that your metabolism decreases, and you may experience low blood sugar, especially if you eat a diet high in sweets. In addition, you may detox too quickly, which is unpleasant and may become a medical issue. Most individuals probably could not or would not attempt a water fast.

During a water-only fast, the bowels cease to move. During a water fast, poisons and toxins are broken down and removed from the bloodstream and intestines. Therefore, an enema is necessary to flush out as much as possible. When ending the water fast, one must gradually reintroduce solid foods into the diet.

There are centers where you can get assistance with water fasting; they monitor your blood levels and guide the process. However, I think water-only fasting for a colon cleanse weight reduction regimen would be the most challenging.

A colon cleanse weight reduction program known as the "Lemon Juice Diet," or "the Maple Syrup Diet," is an additional liquid strategy known as the "Master Cleanse." According to Wikipedia, the Master Cleanse formula was devised by Stanley Burroughs in 1941.

Typically, the Master Cleanse recipe comprises cayenne pepper, distilled water, freshly squeezed lemon juice, and grade B maple syrup. The maple syrup must be authentic maple syrup and not pancake syrup. Also required is sea salt (not regular iodized table salt). The salt is for a colonic saltwater flush. You can also use a herbal laxative to ensure regular bowel movements.

The lemons are believed to alkalize the body, the cayenne pepper assists with circulation, and the maple syrup may be designed to provide minerals and control blood sugar levels. It would help if you weaned yourself off the diet with care.

Don't expect to have a steak meal as soon as you stop this diet. You will need to gradually reintroduce food to your system, beginning with mild broths. This colon cleanse weight reduction treatment lasts between 10 and 30 days. Research this well to ensure you understand what you're doing.

Juice fasting is a safer and more effective alternative to water fasting for colon cleansing and weight reduction plans. However, this plan demands some forethought on your behalf. First, you must juice fresh, organic fruits and vegetables. Juicing does require a certain amount of preparation time.

There is recipe preparation, grocery shopping, produce cleaning, chopping, juicing, and cleaning the juicer machine. You may wish to make a large quantity of juice at once to save time. If you make a large quantity of juice, store it in an airtight container for up to a day.

Also, if you purchase your ingredients in advance, you will not be enticed by the aromas from the deli and bakery and the easy-to-grab candy bars at the checkout counter. Instead, you can choose fruits and vegetables and combine them.

You are not limited to fruits; you may include celery, carrots, cucumbers, and whatever else you like. You can choose nutrient-dense foods such as wheat grass. I must say that a small amount of wheatgrass goes a very long way. You can put spices in your juice.

This colon cleanse weight reduction regimen might be entertaining. Watermelon juice is my favorite flavor. Unlike the water fast, you provide your body with nutrients and assist with blood sugar levels. To remove poisons from the body, you must continue to defecate.

Herbal formulations are utilized in another common colon cleanse and weight loss treatment. There are different formulae available. The herbs and fiber aid in dislodging any stored feces and removing them from the body. Some herbal colon cleanse weight loss remedies require a certain diet, while others only require you to utilize the product.

I've seen cleansing programs that are quite extensive and have a strict daily schedule to adhere to. Ensure you drink plenty of pure water, which is an essential consideration. Some herbal programs include psyllium husks as a source of fiber to remove waste and toxins from the body.

This type of fiber expands significantly when exposed to fluids. A person I spoke with who consumed too much psyllium and did not drink enough water or juice ended up with an intestinal condition. If you use herbal formulae, read and adhere to the recommendations.

Some colon cleanse weight loss regimens use a more thorough cleansing strategy. There are both gluten-free and non-GMO formulations available. They may comprise anti-parasite support formulations or probiotics that aid in the restoration of good intestinal bacteria.

The colon cleansing products are available in the form of tablets, capsules, powders, and teas. If you purchase colon cleansing pills, select the capsules because they dissolve more effectively and quickly than tablets.

A colon cleanse weight reduction regimen can also consist of a series of. You can search for colonic hydrotherapy, colonic irrigation, or colon cleansing to locate a facility that provides these services. This includes flushing the large intestine with water that has been heated to a specific temperature. It is an effective and safe procedure.

A colonoscopy can be somewhat embarrassing. The procedure takes approximately 40 to 50 minutes per session. In my location, the price for each session is approximately $90, but you may be able to purchase multiple sessions at a discount. This can be accomplished without cost by doing an enema at home.

The only required supplies are an enema bag and clean water. When doing an enema, the water should be warm, not hot or cold. Regardless of the colon cleanse weight loss strategy, you may wish to flush the intestines in addition to your herbal or dietary cleanse for optimal results.

What are the hazards associated with a colon cleanse diet? Some herbs and supplements can interfere with or alter the effects of medications. There may be many hazards, and you should visit your doctor, particularly if you have any preexisting medical illnesses or concerns.

When you undergo a colon cleanse weight reduction program, cleansing responses may occur. Depending on your circumstances and toxin load, you may experience mild to severe cleansing effects. You may feel fatigued and have headaches, flu-like symptoms, excessive perspiration, and rashes. During a cleanse, you should avoid excessive exertion and prepare to rest.

Natural Foods to Eat for a Colon Cleanse Detox Diet

While there are many products on the market to assist with a colon cleanse, you can also do it naturally by altering your diet. You can cleanse your system with foods you'll find at your local grocery store. Here is a list of foods you should eat while doing a colon cleanse and detox diet.

Prunes: Prunes are a natural laxative. They also contain vitamin K, antioxidants, dietary fiber, and potassium. In addition, prunes provide your body with beneficial bacteria and enough fiber to keep your colon healthy.

Leafy Green Vegetables: Because they are high in folic acid, vitamin K, dietary fiber, calcium, magnesium, and vitamin C, leafy greens are an essential part of a colon detox diet. In addition, leafy greens contain large amounts of chlorophyll, one of the best nutrients to eat during any detox diet. Arugula, bokchoy, kale, and spinach are a few of the leafy greens you should eat during a colon cleanse.

Apples: Apples are high in fiber and low in fat and calories. Organic apples are best because commercially grown apples are treated with pesticides, and the residue may harm your body. Drinking fresh-squeezed apple juice is another option for good colon health.

Seeds and Nuts: Eating raw seeds and nuts is good for your body during a cleanse because they contain protein, vitamin E, fiber, and other nutrients that your body needs. The best nuts are walnuts, hazelnuts, cashews, almonds, pistachios, and Brazil nuts.

Bananas: Bananas are another good food to eat during a cleanse. They are very portable and contain about 20 percent of the fiber your body needs each day. Bananas are also high in potassium, which helps restore electrolytes in your intestines. In addition, bananas contain fructooligosaccharide, a natural compound that encourages the growth of good bacteria in your intestines.

Tomatoes are a wonderful source of vitamin C, fiber, vitamin K, and vitamin A. They also contain a lot of lycopene, which helps protect your body from developing prostate or colon cancer. Eating organic, locally grown tomatoes benefits your body more than conventionally-grown tomatoes from the grocery store.

Oranges are another portable fruit that is easy to take with you wherever you need to go. They are high in calcium, fiber, vitamin C, and vitamin A. Drinking orange juice is not recommended during a colon cleanse because the juice from an orange doesn't contain enough fiber to assist the natural cleansing process.

Avocados: Avocados are full of nutrients, including folate, vitamin K, dietary fiber, and potassium. One avocado provides your body with about 30 percent of the fiber it needs to function properly for the whole day.

Cranberries are known for their unique ability to prevent and treat urinary tract infections. In addition, these little red berries are great for promoting gastrointestinal health. They contain dietary fiber, vitamin C, and vitamin K, as well as natural probiotics. Cranberries are one of the best foods to eat during a colon cleanse and detox diet. You can eat them fresh or drink cranberry juice as long as no sugar has been added.

By eating a temporary diet of only these foods, you will be able to flush out your colon in no time, naturally. Depending on what you have been eating, your system may take a day to respond. Plan on being flexible with your schedule as you begin a colon cleanse in case you don't feel well as your body adjusts. Keeping a healthy colon and digestive system is important for removing toxins from the body and maintaining overall health.

Eating Habits You Should Follow

Food choices aren't the only factors affecting your gut health. The way you eat and how much you eat can also reveal a lot about how well your digestive track is. If you are a stress eater or you submit yourself to strict dieting, there's a good chance you could be harming your gut.

Never skip your breakfast. As much as it sounds cliché, eating the first meal of the day can improve your gut health right. Aside from giving you the energy you'll need for your daily activities, eating breakfast can also help you avoid unhealthy food choices. Additionally, breakfast prepares your metabolism for your subsequent meals. By warming up your metabolism, you're primarily stimulating it to work more efficiently. Failure to do so, on the other hand, can result in a sluggish ability to metabolize foods, weight gain, and bloating.

Chew your food properly. Breaking down food is already a tedious task for your gut. Improperly chewed foods, meanwhile, are far more strenuous for your digestion. Not only will your gut need to produce more acid, but it will also be forced to work harder to break the pieces effectively. As a result, gulping down food without chewing it properly can result in excessive gas and bloating.

Eat in moderate proportions. Eating too much food in a single meal can cause stomach pain and indigestion. Instead of having three large meals daily, you can break your meals into six small sets. This way, it will be easier for your gut to process the food effectively and efficiently.

Avoid eating right away when you're stressed. Eating when stressed can cause bloating and indigestion. This results from your sympathetic nervous system activating in response to its perceived stress. When this system is triggered, your digestive system shuts down to allow more blood and oxygen to reach the organs necessary for the fight-or-flight response. With less blood on the digestive track, the foods you introduce will not be effectively processed. So instead of working on your plate immediately, take a few deep breaths to calm your system first. Deep breathing is considered effective in managing stress.

Drink enough water. Hydration is essential for your gut health. Drinking enough water daily can help ensure it functions at its best. Water serves as lubrication for your gut. When there is enough lubrication, peristalsis, or food movement through your digestive track, happens smoothly. Hydration, however, does not involve carbonated drinks and fruit juices. These drinks contain too much sugar, which can serve as good food sources for the bad bacteria in your gut.

Listen to your gut. Loose bowel movements, cramping, and bloating are signs of something wrong with your gut. However, it doesn't readily mean that your digestive system suffers from a disease. Most of the time, gut symptoms mean you're doing something wrong. By taking time to understand those symptoms and what their probable causes are, you'll get a good idea of how you'll be able to avoid them permanently.

Constipation

It would help if you tried different things for your constipation story to see what works best for you. Everyone is different. And there are many different kinds of constipation and reasons for having it. If you are throwing up, in terrible pain, or notice blood in your stools, you need to see a doctor because you could have something serious!

Doctors are not always helpful. However, they can give you tests. For example, you could have liver troubles. Or you could have gallstones or liver stones. Or it could be something else that only a doctor is qualified to diagnose. For example, suppose you are just constipated, but you are fully impacted to the point that absolutely nothing can get through your colon. In that case, your doctor can do x-rays to find out how constipated you are, and if you are fully compacted, they'll usually decide to give you a colonoscopy.

They have this super disgusting drink that makes you drink ginormous amounts. This drink will force every poo out of you and clean you out. It's a horrible experience, but afterward you should feel a lot better! And if you are so impacted that even this doesn't work, they will pull all of the poo out of you!

It's gross, and no one wants to be the one to have to do it, but in certain emergencies, it's what's needed. And then you will wake up and feel so much better! It will give you a brand new lease on life, and you can start again with healthier habits and hopefully never suffer from constipation again. Or at least not very often.

You could also try sticking your finger up your butt to see if you can feel any poo and pull it out yourself. If it's too high up, you might not be able to reach it, but if you can feel it in there and it's bothering you, it may be worth a shot.

There are many other things you can try to rid yourself of constipation, and the rest of this book will be dedicated to listing every home remedy I know about.

Leaky Gut Syndrome

Leaky Gut Syndrome affects the lining of the intestines, the first line of defense in the human immune system. The individual epithelial cells that form the outer layer of the intestinal lining are connected by structures called "tight junctures."

The microvilli at the tips of these cells absorb digested nutrients and carry them through the epithelial cells and into the bloodstream, where they nourish the body.

The tight junctures remain closed in a digestive system that is functioning normally. They screen the molecules by only allowing them to pass through the mucosa cells into the bloodstream.

If the tight junctures get stuck in an "open" position, the intestinal lining becomes too porous and cannot perform this filtering process. This allows bacteria, toxins, and partially digested fats and proteins to leak into the bloodstream. When that happens, the body's autoimmune reaction is triggered.

Autoimmune Response to Leaky Gut

As the gut begins to leak, the liver works overtime to take up the slack and screen out the particles coming out of the intestine.

Unfortunately, the flow of waste is more than the liver can handle, and the undigested food, yeast, toxins, and other pathogens begin to accumulate in the body.

Although the immune system continues to wage war on the invaders, tissues throughout the body begin to absorb the material. Once that happens, widespread inflammation develops, stressing the system even more.

The Consequences of Leaky Gut

The longer the gut leaks, the more symptoms the individual experiences. These will likely include gas and bloating, chronic fatigue, joint pain, skin rashes, and growing food sensitivity.

Leaky gut can lead to Crohn's , celiac disease, rheumatoid arthritis, and asthma, or make each of these conditions worse if they are already present. It has further been linked to the following:

- Multiple sclerosis

- Fibromyalgia

- Autism

- Chronic fatigue syndrome

- Eczema

- Dermatitis

- Ulcerative colitis

If any form of inflammatory bowel disease is already present, the person is at a higher risk of developing a leaky gut, which creates a vicious cycle of gastrointestinal issues. If food sensitivities to 8-12 items are present, you likely have a leaky gut and don't even know it.

The Causes of Leaky Gut

The exact cause or causes of leaky gut are up for serious debate, but there seem to be some common and known contributing factors.

- Diet

High levels of refined sugars, processed foods packed with preservatives, refined flours, food dyes, and flavorings are all toxic agents that will increase the degree of inflammation and, thus, permeability in the digestive tract.

- Stress

Ongoing stress is brutal on the body in several ways and is especially hard on the digestive system. Stress suppresses the immune system, which means it cannot efficiently fight pathogens and is subject to being quickly overwhelmed and "outgunned."

- Chronic Inflammation

Inflammation of any sort can lead to a leaky gut. This irritation may be caused by low levels of stomach acid that lead to under digested food passing into the small intestine, resulting in an overgrowth of yeast. Other culprits include bacteria, parasites, environmental toxins, and infections.

- Yeast

Although yeast is a normally occurring flora in the gut, an overgrowth leads to the multi-celled fungus that attaches to the intestinal lining and creates holes.

- Zinc Deficiency

The intestinal lining requires zinc to remain strong. Without proper levels, the lining will weaken and become more subject to developing permeability.

Leaky gut may also result from the overuse of non-steroidal anti-inflammatory drugs, cytotoxic drugs, a course of radiation, certain antibiotics, and excessive alcohol consumption.

- Colonic Cleansing and Leaky Gut

Colonic hydrotherapy and introducing probiotics directly into the colon during the procedure are one of the most effective treatment combinations for healing the intestine and reversing leaky gut syndrome.

Colon cleansing encourages the bowel's natural function. Unlike an enema, hydrotherapy cleans the entire large intestine. As toxins are removed, the tight junctures begin to close again, removing the permeability and allowing nutrients to be absorbed and filtered.

As the lining repairs itself, the action of peristalsis strengthens, and the colon begins to function normally again.

At the same time, all the corollary conditions caused by a leaky gut begin to heal because the liver and immune system can now get ahead of the problem.

Rather than fighting a losing battle against a steady stream of toxins leaking from the intestine, the liver can cleanse the blood as it should, and the immune system can address and correct inflammation in the body.

Goals of a Colon Cleansing Diet

When you concentrate on eating to protect your colon and promote weight loss, you're waging war on all the toxins in the modern food supply.

Many of these materials come from a high concentration of processed items. (Smokers should work on quitting, and alcohol consumption should be limited or eliminated.)

Specific considerations with an eating program of this type include:

An Avoidance of High-fat Foods

Foods that are high in fat contribute to elevated blood pressure and weight gain, two critical factors in the eventual development of heart disease. Examples include potato chips, French fries, anything slathered in butter, organ meats, and pork.

Processed Foods

Items that are canned or frozen contain chemicals and preservatives, but much of their nutritional value is lost. Therefore, it is always better to eat a fresh diet containing no additives or so-called "stabilizers."

Caffeine

Caffeine is very detrimental to colon function because it has a constipating effect. Remember that caffeine doesn't just come from coffee but can also be found in tea, soft drinks, and chocolate.

Sweets and Candy

These items increase the body's insulin production, raising the risk of diabetes. In addition, studies have found that about 76% of patients with diabetes also suffer from some form of gastrointestinal disorder.

Limit Dairy Products

Dairy products are hard to digest, even for those who seem to "tolerate" the items well. Abstaining from or severely limiting dairy intake significantly reduces pressure on the digestive tract.

Above all, aim to drink at least 8 full glasses of water daily. Good hydration is crucial for proper bowel function. Unfortunately, chronic, mild dehydration exists at epidemic levels in the developed world thanks to the over-consumption of soda and coffee.

Specific Colon Cleanse Diets

It's no surprise that the diet section of your local bookstore is bulging with all kinds of books about eating for this or that goal. Colon cleansing is no exception. Often, these plans are mixed with some form of juicing or detoxification.

Beware of any eating program that places long-term and intense demands on your whole body. It would be beneficial if you always considered how any new diet will affect your overall well-being, often in consultation with your doctor or health advisor.

Good Colon Nutrition

By following the basic guidelines of good nutrition for the colon, weight loss will occur naturally over time. Studies have shown that slow and steady weight loss is more sustainable than rapid ups and downs on the scale.

Also, some substances, like gluten, that irritate the gut can take six months or longer to work their way out of your system completely.

Regardless of any diet "program" you might read about or choose to follow, the staples of sound colon health include:

Fruits and Vegetables

In addition to providing fiber, the nutrients in plant-based foods decrease inflammation in the body. In addition, they provide folate, a B-complex vitamin believed to decrease the risk of colon cancer, and they are high in antioxidants.

Whole Grains

Whole grain foods are high in fiber to assist with proper bowel function, and many "fortified" bowls of cereal also contain folate. Be careful, however. A high percentage of cereals are heavily sugared and processed. So make sure you're getting whole grains in healthy foods, not junk food by another name.

Fish

Avoid high-fat meats like pork and red meats high in saturated fats if you eat meat. Opting for fish over these items will lower your risk of colorectal cancer while providing heart-healthy Omega-3.

The More Natural Your Diet, the Better

The more natural, high-fiber foods in your diet, the better. Eating a primarily plant-based diet with limited dairy and meat will not only trim your waistline but also greatly enhance the functioning of the bowel.

A healthy bowel not only allows you to extract necessary nutrients from the foods you eat but also eliminates a prime source of inflammation and opens the door to infections and autoimmune disease.

The weight loss aspect of a colon cleansing diet is certainly attractive, but the long-term health benefits are much more compelling!

Chapter 8: FAQs

While it is highly recommended that you read the entire text to understand how the colon functions in the human gastrointestinal tract and how colonics can enhance that functioning, the following are some of the most commonly asked questions on this topic.

- What is the colon?

Also referred to as the large intestine or bowel, the colon is a five-foot-long tubular passage at the end of the human digestive tract. It measures roughly 2.5 inches (6.35 cm) in diameter.

The colon's function is to eliminate waste material from the body and conserve water. In addition, the bacteria in the colon synthesize nutrients from the food we eat.

- Why do people opt to undergo colon cleansing procedures?

Adherents of colon cleansing believe that our modern lifestyle, which couples high stress levels with a poor diet, is not optimum for efficient digestive performance.

If the colon cannot clear out all the waste material it processes, inflammation, infection, and a host of problems, from simple constipation to colorectal cancer, have a greater chance of becoming established in the bowel.

Colon cleansing supports the natural function of the bowel and promotes overall good health.

- Won't an enema or laxative do the same thing?

Enemas will effectively empty the last 8-12 inches of the colon, called the rectum. Laxatives do the same thing and are useful for alleviating temporary constipation.

Hydrotherapy, however, reaches all areas of the bowel, strengthening the muscles in the process, and promoting more regular, natural bowel movements.

- Are there any added benefits to having a colonic?

Yes. You will work with a trained therapist for 45 minutes to an hour. During that time, you will discuss your diet and lifestyle, exploring other adjustments you can make to support healthy bowel function.

While a colonic treatment empties the bowel of waste thoroughly, the treatment's goal is to better your total health profile.

- Is the colonic procedure painful?

On rare occasions, people do experience mild cramping during a colonic. However, these episodes pass quickly and are not difficult to tolerate.

Therapists are trained to put their clients at ease and are ready to answer any questions or concerns. Mention any discomfort immediately.

- Isn't a colonic just a little too embarrassing?

The procedure is conducted in a private room with a trained therapist whose job is not only to administer the therapy but to put you at ease and preserve your dignity.

You will be covered at all times, and the parts of the procedure people dread most, including any odor, do not occur because the colonic apparatus is a closed system.

- What should I do to get ready for a colonic irrigation session?

Eat or drink for a couple of hours very lightly before the procedure. There is no need to fast or make any major adjustments to your normal routine.

- Should I do anything special after the procedure is over?

Over a few hours, you may have more bowel movements, but these are not uncomfortable or uncontrollable in terms of urgency. Just carry on with your normal routine.

- Is there any danger involved in colonic hydrotherapy?

When working with a trained therapist in a professional environment where the equipment is properly cleaned and sterilized, there is virtually no danger to this therapy whatsoever.

- I've heard getting colonics is habit-forming. Is this true?

This is a myth. The goal of the therapy is a colon that functions properly. After the procedure, it may take a while for the next bowel movement to occur, which leads some people to think they have become dependent on the procedure to eliminate.

With dietary and lifestyle changes to support colon health, however, better regularity of function is almost assured.

- Will colonic hydrotherapy lead to constipation or diarrhea?

Typically, there will be a delay before the next bowel movement after a colonic session. The stool is generally larger and easier to move when it does occur. Any instance of diarrhea is very rare and short-lived.

- I have been suffering from constipation. Will colonic cleansing help?

For your colon to function properly, you must have a good balance of nutrition and hydration, physical exercise, and emotional well-being. Then, the colonic will clear out the bowel sufficiently to allow the other factors to be adjusted in a much more physically relaxed state.

- I've read that colonics eliminate all the beneficial intestinal bacteria and rob the system of nutrients. Is any of that true?

The bacteria your intestine needs to function can only grow in a balanced environment. Therefore, they live on the colon's wall and are not removed during colonic hydrotherapy.

Suppose there is reason to believe that the bacteria in your bowels are out of balance. In that case, the therapist may implant a post-treatment probiotic or suggest you begin a course of probiotic treatment to correct the issue.

- Does colon cleansing benefit the immune system?

Recent studies completed in Europe have found that as much as 80% of the immune tissue in the human body resides in the intestines.

Since hydrotherapy promotes a healthy colon and works to reduce inflammation, it also serves to protect the immune function of the bowel.

- How soon after giving birth can I have a colonic?

Wait 10-12 weeks after normal childbirth to have a colonic; longer if the birth is difficult or a C-section is required. This is because the body needs a chance to recover, and any stitches must be removed completely. Nursing mothers can have colonics without ill effects on themselves or their children.

- How many bowel movements should I have in a day?

Have you ever wondered why an infant eats her meal and passes stool within minutes of it? The infant is not passing the meal she just ate, but the one she ate an hour ago. This is an example of a perfectly healthy bowel movement; that is how it should be for adults.

We should pass stool within half an hour of our meal. If not, then at least 2-3 bowel movements a day are an absolute must. Unfortunately, our lifestyle and poor diet cause us to have just one bowel movement a day or, worse, a constipated one.

- Why is the size of my bowel movement important?

Our colon is two and a ½ inches round in size. Therefore, our bowel size should be around 2 inches round. A bowel size much bigger or smaller than this size is a sign of a colon problem like constipation.

- What is constipation?

Constipation means irregularity in stools. This irregularity may mean irregular timing or an irregular constituency. Constipated stools are hardened due to a lack of water. Passing them causes pain and can even cause bleeding from the anal walls.

- What causes constipation?

Constipation is caused by factors such as insufficient fluid consumption, insufficient fiber consumption, and insufficient physical activity. Illness, pregnancy, or changes in diet can also lead to constipation. In addition, many over-the-counter medications for coughs and antacids and prescribed medicines for cholesterol and depression can also cause constipation.

- How can I check to see if I am consuming enough fiber?

Everybody has their own requirement for daily fiber. However, with just a few simple observations, you can better understand if you have enough fiber in your diet.

If your diet is fiber-rich, you can expel stools smoothly from your body. As a result, you will not feel pain, and you won't have to apply pressure while passing the bowel.

When a fiber-rich diet is digested, it makes the whole food airy. When you pass such an 'airy' stool, it floats on top of the water and even breaks down quickly in the water itself. In contrast, a diet lacking in fiber is like a sticky, heavy clump that sinks to the toilet bowl's bottom.

- My bowel movement often carries a horrid smell. What does it mean?

A bowel movement with an unbearable odor indicates that the waste was lying in your colon for too long, for more than 24 hours at least. This is extremely unhealthy.

- How much time should I set aside for the procedure?

On your first visit with a therapist, 15 to 30 minutes will be taken to fill out forms and discuss your medical history. After that, the duration of the treatment varies by individual but typically takes about 34 minutes. So for your first appointment, set aside at least two hours.

- Is it alright to eat after a colonic?

Have a regular meal at the time you normally eat. Don't overeat; try to consume something gentle and nourishing to your system.

- I have a problem skin. Will colon cleansing help?

Since your skin is also an important organ for eliminating waste, it stands to reason that toxicity anywhere in the system will cause the skin to suffer. In many cases, clients find that colon cleansing benefits their problem skin.

- How many colon cleansing treatments will I need?

Although most people feel a definite improvement in their sense of wellbeing after a single treatment, changes in diet and lifestyle are necessary to achieve a healthy digestive system.

If you have a long-standing condition, assessing how many treatments will be required isn't easy. However, if you opt for a maintenance program of therapy, the period in between the session will grow longer as your bowel health optimizes.

- Will colon cleansing help me to lose weight?

You will feel lighter after a colonic treatment. There may be some weight loss, but the real improvement will be evident when you take in more fiber, increase your level of exercise, and drink more water.

While these things support good bowel function, they also contribute to safe and permanent weight loss.

- Should colonics be administered during pregnancy?

Typically colonics should not be administered during pregnancy unless a qualified medical practitioner performs the procedure.

Chapter 9: Anti-inflammatory recipes

Lemon and Dates Barramundi

Preparation time: 10 minutes

Cooking time: 12 minutes

Servings: 2

Ingredients

2 barramundi fillets, boneless

One shallot, sliced

Four lemon slices

Juice of ½ lemon

Zest of 1 lemon, grated

2 tbsp. olive oil

6 oz. baby spinach

¼ C. almonds, chopped

Four dates, pitted and chopped

¼ C. parsley, chopped

Salt and black pepper to the taste

Directions

Season the fish with salt and pepper and arrange it on two pieces of parchment paper.

Top the fish with the lemon slices, drizzle the lemon juice, and then top with the other ingredients except for the oil.

Drizzle 1 tbsp. Oil over each fish mix, wrap the parchment paper around the fish, shape them into packets, and arrange them on a baking sheet.

Bake at 400°F for 12 minutes. Cool the mix, unfold it, divide everything between plates, and serve.

Nutrition

Calories: 232 kcal

Fat: 16.5 g

Fiber: 11.1 g

Carbs: 24.8 g

Protein: 6.5 g

Catfish Fillets and Rice

Preparation time: 10 minutes

Cooking time: 55 minutes

Servings: 2

Ingredients

Two catfish fillets, boneless

2 tbsp. Italian seasoning

2 tbsp. olive oil

For the rice:

1 C. brown rice

2 tbsp. olive oil

1 and ½ C. water

½ C. green bell pepper, chopped

2 garlic cloves, minced

½ C. white onion, chopped

2 tsp. Cajun seasoning

½ tsp. garlic powder

Salt and black pepper to the taste

Directions

Heat a pot with 2 tbsp. Oil over medium heat, add the onion, garlic, garlic powder, salt, and pepper, and sauté for 5 minutes.

Add the rice, water, bell pepper, and seasoning; bring to a simmer; and cook over medium heat for 40 minutes.

Heat a pan with 2 tbsp. Oil over medium heat, add the fish and the Italian seasoning, and cook for 5 minutes on each side.

Divide the rice between plates, add the fish on top, and serve.

Nutrition

Calories: 261 kcal

Fat: 17.6 g

Fiber: 12.2 g

Carbs: 24.8 g

Protein: 12.5 g

Halibut Pan

Preparation time: 10 minutes

Cooking time: 20 minutes

Servings: 4

Ingredients

4 halibut fillets, boneless

1 red bell pepper, chopped

2 tbsp. olive oil

1 yellow onion, chopped

4 garlic cloves, minced

½ C. chicken stock

1 tsp. basil, dried

½ C. cherry tomatoes halved

⅓ C. Kalamata olives pitted and halved

Salt and black pepper to the taste

Directions

Heat a pan with the oil over medium heat, add the fish, cook for 5 minutes on each side, and divide between plates.

Add the onion, bell pepper, garlic, and tomatoes to the pan, stir, and sauté for 3 minutes.

Add salt, pepper, and the rest of the ingredients; toss; cook for 3 minutes more; divide next to the fish and serve.

Nutrition

Calories: 253 kcal

Fat: 8 g

Fiber: 1 g

Carbs: 5 g

Protein: 28 g

Baked Shrimp Mix

Preparation time: 10 minutes

Cooking time: 32 minutes

Servings: 4

Ingredients

4 gold potatoes, peeled and sliced

2 fennel bulbs, trimmed and cut into wedges

2 shallots, chopped

2 garlic cloves, minced

3 tbsp. olive oil

½ C. Kalamata olives pitted and halved

2 lb. shrimp, peeled and deveined

1 tsp. lemon zest, grated

2 tsp. oregano, dried

4 oz. feta cheese, crumbled

2 tbsp. parsley, chopped

Directions

In a roasting pan, combine the potatoes with 2 tbsp. Oil, garlic, and the rest of the ingredients, except the shrimp, are tossed, introduced in the oven, and baked at 450°F for 25 minutes.

Add the shrimp, toss, and bake for 7 minutes; divide between plates and serve.

Nutrition

Calories: 341 kcal

Fat: 19 g

Fiber: 9 g

Carbs: 34 g

Protein: 10 g

Shrimp and Lemon Sauce

Preparation time: 10 minutes

Cooking time: 15 minutes

Servings: 4

Ingredients

1 lb. shrimp, peeled and deveined

⅓ C. lemon juice

4 egg yolks

2 tbsp. olive oil

1 C. chicken stock

Salt and black pepper to the taste

1 C. black olives, pitted and halved

1 tbsp. thyme, chopped

Directions

Mix the lemon juice with the egg yolks in a bowl and whisk well.

Heat up a pan with the oil over medium heat, add the shrimp, cook for 2 minutes on each side, and transfer to a plate.

Heat a pan with the stock over medium heat; add some of this over the egg yolks and lemon juice mix and whisk well.

Add this over the rest of the stock; also add salt and pepper; whisk well, and simmer for 2 minutes.

Add the shrimp and the rest of the ingredients, toss, and serve immediately.

Nutrition

Calories: 237 kcal

Fat: 15.3 g

Fiber: 4.6 g

Carbs: 15.4 g

Protein: 7.6 g

Fruit and Yogurt Parfait

Preparation time: 10 minutes

Cooking time: 0 minutes

Servings: 2

Ingredients

2 C. yogurt, lactose-free plain, non-fat

3 tbsp. pure maple syrup

¼ tsp. ginger, ground

½ banana, peeled and sliced

¼ C. pecans, chopped

Directions

Whisk together the yogurt, syrup, and ginger in a small bowl.

Spoon ½ C. of the yogurt mixture into each of the 2 parfait glasses.

Top each with ½ of the banana slices.

Top each with another ½ C. yogurt mixture.

Sprinkle each with 2 tbsp. Pecans. Serve.

Nutrition

Calories: 354 kcal

Protein: 14 g

Fat: 14 g

Carbs: 46 g

Maple-Ginger Oatmeal

Preparation time: 5 minutes

Cooking time: 0 minutes

Servings: 2

Ingredients

1½ C. water

Pinch salt

1 C. oats, old-fashioned, rolled

¼ C. pure maple syrup

½ tsp. ginger, ground

Directions

Bring the water and salt to a boil over medium-high heat in a small pot.

Stir in the oats, syrup, and ginger.

Reduce the heat to medium-low. Cook, frequently stirring, for 5 minutes. Serve.

Nutrition

Calories: 258 kcal

Protein: 7 g

Fat: 3 g

Carbs: 53 g

Corn Porridge With Maple and Raisins

Preparation time: 5 minutes

Cooking time: 0 minutes

Servings: 2

Ingredients

¾ C. cornmeal

2¼ C. water, divided

Pinch salt

1 tbsp. pure maple syrup

3 tbsp. raisins

Directions

In a small mixing bowl, combine the cornmeal and 34 cup of water.

In a small pot, bring the remaining 1½ C. of water and the salt to a boil over medium-high heat.

Whisk in the cornmeal slurry. Cook, stirring frequently, for 10–12 minutes, until thick.

Stir in the maple syrup and raisins. Then serve hot.

Nutrition

Calories: 288 kcal

Protein: 6 g

Fat: 3 g

Carbs: 60 g

Milky Oat

Preparation time: 8 minutes

Cooking time: 0 minutes

Servings: 2

Ingredients

1 C. oats

½ C. coconut milk, low-fat

½ C. water

1 tsp. liquid stevia

Directions

Mix together the coconut milk and water in the saucepan.

Add the oats and stir.

Close the lid and cook the oats over medium heat for 10 minutes.

Let them chill for 5–10 minutes when the oats are cooked.

Then add liquid stevia and stir it.

After this, transfer the milky oats to the bowls and serve!

Nutrition

Calories: 293 kcal

Fat: 17 g

Carbs: 31 g

Protein: 6.8 g

Chia Breakfast

Preparation time: 15 minutes

Cooking time: 0 minutes

Servings: 4

Ingredients

1 ½ C. quinoa

2 ½ C. water

8 tbsp. chia seeds

2 C. low-fat hemp milk

1 date, pitted

1 tbsp. almonds, chopped

1 tbsp. coconut, shredded

Directions

Pour water into the pan and add quinoa.

Close the lid and cook for 15 minutes.

When the quinoa is cooked, chill it a little.

After this, place the hemp milk and pitted dates in the blender.

Blend the mixture until smooth and transfer to a big bowl.

Add chia seeds and stir well.

After this, leave the mixture for 10 minutes more.

Then add cooked quinoa. Stir it.

Transfer the cooked breakfast to the serving bowls.

Sprinkle the meal with chopped almonds and shredded coconut.

Enjoy!

Nutrition

Calories: 453 kcal

Fat: 17.3 g

Carbs: 60 g

Protein: 16.7 g

Apple Parfait

Preparation time: 10 minutes

Cooking time: 0 minutes

Servings: 2

Ingredients

2 oz. cashews, soaked

2 oz. low-fat coconut milk

¼ tsp. vanilla extract

2 apples, chopped

1 tbsp. hemp seeds

Directions

Place the cashews, coconut milk, vanilla extract, and hemp seeds into the blender.

Blend the mixture until smooth and homogenous.

After this, place a small amount of the smooth mixture into the glass.

Then make a layer of chopped apples.

Repeat the layers until you have put in all the ingredients.

Serve it!

Nutrition

Calories: 367 kcal

Fat: 22 g

Carbs: 42 g

Protein: 6.8 g

Mexican Breakfast Toast

Preparation time: 5 minutes

Cooking time: 20 minutes

Servings: 2

Ingredients

2 slices sprouted bread, toasted

2 tbsp. hummus

½ C. spinach, chopped

¼ red onion, sliced

½ C. sprouts

1 avocado, thinly sliced

¼ tsp. Himalayan salt

Spicy Yogurt

3 tbsp. yogurt, unsweetened

½ lime, juiced

1 tsp. cumin

1 tsp. cayenne

Directions

In a small bowl, prepare the spicy yogurt by combining all the ingredients and whisking well to combine.

Place toast slices on plates and spread a tbsp. of hummus on each. Place spinach on each slice, and then spicy yogurt, red onion, sprouts, and avocado. Sprinkle each with salt and serve.

Nutrition

Calories: 438 kcal

Carbohydrates: 15 g

Protein: 23 g

Fat: 36 g

Saturated Fat: 12 g

Sodium: 1457 mg

Fiber: 3 g

Chapter 10: Vegan recipes

Quinoa

Preparation time: 15 minutes

Cooking time: 20 minutes

Servings: 2–4

Ingredients

1 C. quinoa

3 scallions, chopped

¼ green bell pepper, chopped

½ plum tomato, chopped

1 ½ C. water

¼ tsp. sea salt

⅛ tsp. thyme

dash cayenne pepper

Directions

Submerge the quinoa for 5 minutes, strain, and rinse to remove wax. Add all the ingredients to a saucepan and bring to a boil.

Lower the heat, then simmer until the water is absorbed.

Nutrition

Calories:120 kcal

Protein:4.4 g

Fiber: 2.8 g

Kale Wraps With Chili, Garlic, Cucumber, Coriander, and Green Beans

Preparation time: 30 minutes

Cooking time: 20 minutes

Servings: 1

Ingredients

1 tbsp. fresh lime juice

1 tbsp. raw seed mix

2 kale leaves

2 tsp. fresh garlic

½ avocado, ripe

1 tsp. fresh red chili

1 C. fresh cucumber sticks

½ C. fresh coriander leaves

1 C. green beans

Directions

Spread kale leaves on a clean kitchen work surface. Next, spread each chopped coriander leaf on each lea, and position them around the end of the leaf, perpendicular to the edge.

Spread green beans equally on each leaf, at the edge of each leaf, the same as the coriander leaves. Do the same thing with the cucumber sticks.

Cut the divided, chopped garlic across each leaf, sprinkling it all over the green beans. Next, cut and spread the chopped chili across each leaf and sprinkle it over the garlic. Now, divide the avocado across each leaf and spread it over the chili, garlic, coriander, and green beans.

Share the raw seed mix among each leaf and sprinkle it over other ingredients. Next, divide the lime juice across each leaf and drizzle it over all the other ingredients.

Now, fold or roll up the kale leaves and wrap up all the ingredients. Finally, you can serve it with soy sauce!

Nutrition

Calories:305 kcal

Fiber:18 g

Protein:30 g

Cabbage Wraps With Avocado

Preparation time: 30 minutes

Cooking time: 15 minutes

Servings: 1

Ingredients

½ C. raw pecan nuts

½ C. fresh strawberries, sliced

2 cabbage leaves

½ avocado, ripe

1 C. green asparagus spears

Directions

Spread out the cabbage sheets on a clean kitchen work surface. Share the asparagus shear among each cabbage leaf and place them on the edge of the leaf. Next, share the avocado slices on each leaf and put them on the asparagus spears.

Share the strawberries over each leaf and spread them on top of the avocado slices. Next, share the pecan nuts between each leaf and spread them on the strawberries.

Wrap the leaves with all the ingredients inside them. Serve with soy sauce (optional).

Nutrition

Calories:119 kcal

Fiber:13 g

Protein: 31 g

Millet Tabbouleh, Lime, and Cilantro

Preparation time: 10 minutes

Cooking time: 30 minutes

Servings: 6

Ingredients

½ C. lime juice

½ C. cilantro

6 drops of hot sauce

¼ C. and 2 tsp. olive oil

2 tomatoes

2 green onions

2 cucumbers

1 C. millet

Directions

Heat the olive oil in a saucepan over medium heat. Add the millet and fry until it begins to smell fragrant (which takes 3–4 minutes). Add about 6 c. of water and bring to a boil.

Wait for about 15 minutes. Then, turn off the heat, wash, and rinse under cold water. Finally, drain the millet and transfer it to a large bowl.

Add cucumbers, tomatoes, lime juice, cilantro, green onions, ¼ C. oil, and hot sauce. Season with pepper and salt to taste.

Nutrition

Calories:211 kcal

Fiber:15 g

Protein: 30 g

Alkaline Cauliflower Fried Rice With Kale, Ginger, And Turmeric

Preparation time: 5 minutes

Cooking time: 5 minutes

Servings: 4

Ingredients

1 lime

4 spring onions

2 almonds

1 tbsp. coconut oil

1 large cauliflower

1 bunch mint

1-inch fresh root turmeric

1 Courgette zucchini

½ bunch kale

1 cauliflower

1 tsp. tamari soy sauce

½ bunch parsley

Directions

First, cut the cauliflower into smaller florets and blend them in a food processor or blender. Process it until it begins to look like rice. Next, prep the veggies. Roughly chop off the herbs like parsley, mint, and coriander.

Throw away the parsley and mint stems, but keep them off the coriander. Slice the courgettes and kale thinly. Peel off the turmeric and ginger, then grate both into a pan containing coconut oil. Once it gets warm, stir the mint, parsley, coriander, and coriander stem into the mix.

Wait for thirty seconds and stir in the kale and cauliflower. After two to three minutes, add the tamari, spring onions, and the remaining herbs. Stir properly and turn off the heat.

Lastly, chop the almonds and stir through. Season to taste and sprinkle lime.

Nutrition

Calories:304 kcal

Fiber:14 g

Protein:33 g

Alkaline Salad With Mint and Lemon Toppings

Preparation time: 15 minutes

Cooking time: 20 minutes

Servings: 4

Ingredients

200 g green peas

5 radishes

½ bunch cilantro

Avocado, sliced

3 asparagus

½ bunch flat leaf parsley

2 Courgette zucchinis

For the dressing:

2 shallots

3 lemons

15 g Dijon mustard

1 garlic clove

190 ml olive oil

Black pepper and Himalayan salt to taste

¼ bunch mint

Directions

First of all, let's start with asparagus. First, boil water in a pan; when it gets to the boiling point, immerse the asparagus inside for about 1 minute.

Remove it and rinse immediately in cold water. After that, slice it into long strips. Next, get a frying pan and fry the zucchini over medium heat until it turns brown.

Mix the cilantro, radish, parsley, peas, avocado, asparagus, and zucchini in a large bowl. To make the dressing, blend all ingredients into a food processor—dress and season.

Nutrition

Calories:258 kcal

Fiber:17 g

Protein:28 g

Alkaline Sushi-Roll Ups

Preparation time: 15 minutes

Cooking time: 20 minutes

Servings: 2

Ingredients

For hummus:

1 garlic clove

½ lemon juice

Handful almonds

1 pinch cumin

1 pinch of Himalayan salt

A glug of olive oil

1 tsp. tahini

100 g chickpeas

For the roll-ups:

1 cucumber

2 zucchini/Courgette

1 carrot

1 capsicum

1 small coriander/cilantro

1 avocado

Directions

For the Hummus:

All you have to do is get a food processor or blender. Then, blend until everything is smooth.

Then add some more lemon or olive oil to suit your taste.

For the alkaline sushi roll-ups:

Cut off both ends of the zucchini. Then, use a vegetable peeler to peel it into thin, long strips.

Layout the zucchini strips and spread the almond hummus on them.

Add some matchsticks of avocado, some veggies, and a few pieces of coriander. Spray some of the sesame seeds on top. Roll and enjoy.

Nutrition

Calories:158 kcal

Fiber:10 g

Fats: 9 g

Tabbouleh Salad

Preparation time: 20 minutes

Cooking time: 15 minutes

Servings: 4

Ingredients

2 C. water, filtered

1 C. millet, rinsed

⅓ C. extra-virgin olive oil

Juice of 1 lemon

1 large garlic clove, crushed

1½ tsp. Himalayan pink salt, divided

2 large tomatoes, rinsed and finely diced

3 scallions, white parts only, rinsed and thinly sliced

½ English cucumber, rinsed and finely diced

¾ C. fresh mint, rinsed and finely chopped

1½ C. fresh parsley, rinsed and finely chopped

Directions

Boil water over high heat. Add the millet and turn the heat to low. Cover the pan and cook for 15 minutes.

Remove the pan from the heat and mash the millet with a fork. Allow to cool for 15 minutes with the lid off . It should be firm but not crunchy or mushy.

Meanwhile, in a small bowl, whisk the olive oil, lemon juice, garlic, and ½ tsp. of salt. Let sit.

In a large bowl, combine the tomatoes, scallions, cucumber, mint, and parsley. Add the cooled millet. Pour the dressing on the salad and mix well;taste and season with the remaining 1 tsp. of salt, as needed.

Nutrition

Calories:360 kcal

TotalFat:20 g

TotalCarbohydrates:44 g

Fiber:8 g

Sugar:3 g

Protein:8 g

Guacamole Salad

Preparation time: 10 minutes

Cooking time: 0 minute

Servings: 2

Ingredients

2 avocados, halved and pitted

½ C. red onion, diced

½ C. fresh cilantro, rinsed and chopped

Juice of ½ lime

½ tsp. onion powder

½ tsp. cayenne, ground

½ tsp. Himalayan pink salt

1 tomato, rinsed and diced

Directions

Take out the avocado flesh and place it in a medium bowl. Stir in the red onion, cilantro, lime juice, onion powder, cayenne, and salt. Mash everything until it's smooth. Add the tomato, mix well, and serve.

Nutrition

Calories:450 kcal

TotalFat:40 g

TotalCarbohydrates:27 g

Fiber:16 g

Buckwheat Salad

Preparation time: 10 minutes

Cooking time: 15 minutes

Servings: 2

Ingredients

1 C. raw buckwheat, rinsed

2 C. water

2 handfuls fresh baby spinach leaves, rinsed

Handful fresh basil leaves, rinsed

2 scallions, white parts only, rinsed and chopped

Zest of 1 lemon

Juice of ½ lemon

½ red onion, finely chopped

Himalayan pink salt

Black pepper, freshly ground

¼ C. extra-virgin olive oil

1 red chili, rinsed and thinly sliced

2 tbsp. mixed sprouts, rinsed

1 ripe avocado, peeled, pitted, and sliced

1½ oz. feta cheese (optional)

Directions

Mix the buckwheat and water, then bring it to a boil over high heat. Reduce the heat to simmer and cook for 15 minutes or until soft. Remove from the heat and set aside to cool..

Meanwhile, in a food processor, combine the baby spinach, basil, scallions, lemon zest, and lemon juice and process for 30 seconds. Stir the herb mixture into the cooled buckwheat.

Add the red onion and season with salt and pepper. Arrange the buckwheat on a platter. Drizzle with the olive oil and scatter on the chopped chili and sprouts. Top with the sliced avocado, crumble the feta over the top (if using), and serve.

Nutrition

Calories:685 kcal

TotalFat:54 g

TotalCarbohydrates:43 g

Fiber:16 g

Sugar:5 g

Mixed Sprouts Salad

Preparation time: 10 minutes

Cooking time: 0 minute

Servings: 2

Ingredients

1–2 tbsp. coconut oil

Juice of 1 lemon

A handful of fresh chives, rinsed and chopped

A handful of fresh dill, rinsed and chopped

A handful of fresh parsley, rinsed and chopped

½ tsp. Himalayan pink salt

½ tsp. black pepper, freshly ground

1 scallion, rinsed and chopped

1 cucumber, rinsed and chopped

½ C. mixed sprouts of choice (alfalfa, radish, broccoli, mung bean, cress, etc.), rinsed

Directions

In a blender, combine the coconut oil, lemon juice, chives, dill, parsley, salt, and pepper, and blend until mostly smooth. Transfer to a medium bowl. Stir in the scallion, cucumber, and sprouts to coat, and serve.

Nutrition

Calories:168 kcal

TotalFat:14 g

TotalCarbohydrates:12 g

Fiber:1 g

Sugar:4 g

Thai Quinoa Salad

Preparation time: 15 minutes

Cooking time: 0 minute

Servings: 2

Ingredients

For the dressing:

⅓ C. water, filtered

¼ C. tahini

1 date, pitted

1 tbsp. sesame seeds

1 tbsp. apple cider vinegar

2 tsp. tamari

1 tsp. lemon juice, freshly squeezed

1 tsp. sesame oil, toasted

1 tsp. Garlic, chopped

½ tsp. Himalayan pink salt

For the salad:

1 C. quinoa, rinsed and steamed

1 C. arugula, rinsed and chopped

1 tomato, rinsed and sliced

¼ red onion, rinsed and diced

Directions

To make the dressing:

Blend the water, tahini, dates, sesame seeds, vinegar, tamari, lemon juice, sesame oil, garlic, and salt at high speed until smooth.

To make the salad:

Combine the quinoa, arugula, tomato, and red onion. Drizzle the dressing, toss it well to coat, and serve.

Nutrition

Calories:558 kcal

TotalFat:25 g

TotalCarbohydrates:69 g

Fiber:10 g

Sugar:4 g

Protein:19 g

Sweet Potato Salad

Preparation time: 15 minutes

Cooking time: 5 minutes

Servings: 2

Ingredients

For the dressing:

½ C. sesame oil

2 tbsp. coconut oil

2 tbsp. light soy sauce

1 tbsp. coconut sugar or raw honey

1 garlic clove, crushed

For the salad:

5 ½ oz. fresh baby spinach leaves, rinsed

1 red onion, rinsed and finely chopped

One tomato, rinsed, seeded, and chopped

1 tbsp. coconut oil

1 large sweet potato, scrubbed, peeled, and diced

Directions

To make the dressing:

In a small bowl, whisk the sesame oil, coconut oil, soy sauce, coconut sugar, and garlic until blended. Set aside.

To make the salad:

In a large salad bowl, gently toss the baby spinach, red onion, and tomato. Set aside.

In a small skillet over medium heat, heat the coconut oil. Add the sweet potato and cook for 3–5 minutes, stirring, until golden brown. Add the sweet potato to the salad using a slotted spoon and gently stir to combine. Pour the dressing over the salad, gently toss again to coat, and serve.

Nutrition

Calories:550 kcal

TotalFat:52 g

TotalCarbohydrates:20 g

Fiber:3 g

Sugar:9 g

Chapter 11: Smoothie and juice recipes

Banana kale smoothie

Preparation time: 5 minutes

Cooking time: 10 minutes

Servings: 2

Ingredients:

2 cups kale leaves

1 cup almond milk

½ cup crushed ice

1 banana, peeled

1 apple, peeled and cored

A dash of cinnamon

Directions:

Place all ingredients in a blender.

Blend until smooth.

Pour into a glass container and chill in the fridge for at least 30 minutes.

Nutrition: 165; carbs: 32.1g; Protein: 2.3g; fat: 4.2g Cholesterol: 0mg

Clean green juice

Preparation time: 10 minutes

Cooking time: 0 minutes

Servings: 2

Ingredients

2½ c. Fresh spinach

Two large celery stalks

Two large green apples, cored and sliced

1 medium orange, peeled, seeded, and sectioned

1 tbsp. Fresh lime juice

1 tbsp. Fresh lemon juice

Directions

In a juicer, add all ingredients and extract the juice according to the manufacturer's directions.

Transfer into two serving glasses and stir in lime and lemon juices.

Serve immediately.

Nutrition: Calories 476, fat 40, fiber 9, carbs 33, protein 6

Green tea purifying smoothie

Preparation time: 10 minutes

Cooking time: 0 minutes

Servings: 2

Ingredients

2 c. Fresh baby spinach

3 c. Frozen green grapes

1 medium ripe avocado peeled, pitted, and chopped

2 tsp. Organic honey

1½ c. Strong-brewed green tea

Directions

Put all ingredients in a blender, and blend until smooth.

Transfer into serving glasses and serve immediately.

Nutrition: Calories 476, fat 40, fiber 9, carbs 33, protein 6

Cleansing smoothie

Preparation time: 10 minutes

Cooking time: 0 minutes

Servings: 2

Ingredients:

1 cup water

½ cup papaya chunks

¼ cup organic pineapple chunks

1 teaspoon anti-parasitic coconut oil

1 teaspoon raw pumpkin seeds

A pinch of garlic paste

Directions:

In a blender, combine all of the ingredients until well combined; add ice if desired, and more water if the consistency is too thick to drink easily.

Nutrition: Calories 476, fat 40, fiber 9, carbs 33, protein 6 Cholesterol: 90mg

Blue breeze shake

Preparation time: 10 minutes

Cooking time: 0 minutes

Servings: 2

Ingredients:

½ cup blueberries

1 small banana

1 cup chilled unsweetened vanilla almond milk

Water as needed

1 scoop unflavored protein powder

Directions:

Mix in a blender for 40-50 seconds and serve as ready.

Nutrition: Calories 69, fat 6.5 g, fiber 2.6 g, carbs 10.6 g, protein 9.4 g Cholesterol: 78mg

Citrus mocktail

Preparation time: 10 minutes

Cooking time: 0 minutes

Servings: 2

Ingredients

3 lime slices

11-12 fresh mint leaves plus more for garnishing

6 oz. Lime-flavored seltzer water

1 tbsp. Organic honey

Ice cubes, as required

Directions

In a tall glass, place lime slices and mint leaves, and with a spoon, muddle for about 1 minute.

Add seltzer water, honey, and ice and stir to blend well.

Garnish with mint leaves and serve.

Nutrition: Calories 69, fat 6.5 g, fiber 2.6 g, carbs 10.6 g, protein 9.4 g Cholesterol: 98mg

Coconut breezy shake dose

Preparation time: 10 minutes

Cooking time: 0 minutes

Servings: 2

Ingredients:

1 cup skimmed milk (chilled)

1 cup pineapple chunks

4 tablespoons shredded coconut

Water as needed

½ scoop of vanilla protein powder

Directions:

Put all the ingredients in a mixer and shake well for 20 seconds; serve when the smooth texture is visible. Pour in a large glass and use water to make it smooth.

Nutrition: Calories 476, fat 40, fiber 9, carbs 33, protein 6 Cholesterol: 78mg

Coconut breezy shake dose

Preparation time: 10 minutes

Cooking time: 0 minutes

Servings: 2

Ingredients:

1 cup skimmed milk (chilled)

1 cup pineapple chunks

4 tablespoons shredded coconut

Water as needed

½ scoop of vanilla protein powder

Directions:

Put all the ingredients in a mixer and shake well for 20 seconds; serve when the smooth texture is visible. Pour in a large glass and use water to make it smooth.

Nutrition: Calories 476, fat 40, fiber 9, carbs 33, protein 6 Cholesterol: 78mg

Detoxifying turmeric tea

Preparation 2 minutes

Cooking time 0 minutes

Servings: 4

Ingredients:

1 ½ cups boiling water

One bag of chamomile tea

One bag of peppermint tea

½ teaspoon vanilla extract

One teaspoon turmeric

1 teaspoon ginger

1/4 teaspoon pepper

One teaspoon raw honey

Directions:

In a large mug, combine hot water, chamomile, and peppermint teas and let steep for at least 3 minutes; stir in the remaining ingredients and serve hot!

Nutrition: Calories 100, fat 1, fiber 2, carbs 2, protein 6 Cholesterol: 98mg

Fresh ginger lemonade

Preparation time: 10 minutes

Cooking time: 0 minutes

Servings: 2

Ingredients

2 medium fresh rosemary sprigs

2 tbsp. Fresh ginger root, peeled and grated

4 large lemon peel strips

1/3 c. Organic honey

8 c. Water divided

Fresh juice of 4 lemons

Ice cubes, as required

Lemon slices for garnishing

Directions

In a pan, add rosemary sprigs, ginger, lemon peel strips, honey, and 2 c. of water and bring to a boil.

Reduce the heat to low and simmer for about 10 minutes, stirring continuously.

Remove from the heat and set aside for about 15 minutes to cool.

Through a strainer, strain the mixture into a large pitcher, discarding the solids.

Add the remaining water and lemon juice and stir to blend well.

Pour the lemonade into glasses with ice..

Garnish with lemon slices and serve.

Nutrition: Calories 140, fat 4, fiber 2, carbs 7, protein 8 Cholesterol: 89mg

Ginger citrus liver detox drink

Preparation time: 10 minutes

Cooking time: 0 minutes

Servings: 1

Ingredients

1 lemon, peeled

1-inch knob of fresh ginger root, finely grated

1 orange, peeled

1 grapefruit, peeled

A pinch of cayenne pepper

Directions

Juice all the ingredients in a juicer, except cayenne pepper; stir in cayenne pepper and serve.

Nutrition:

Calories: 11;

Total fat: 0 g;

Carbs: 0 g;

Dietary fiber: 0 g;

Sugars: 1 g;

Protein: 5 g;

Cholesterol: 0 mg;

Sodium: 2 mg

Ginger honey lemonade

Preparation 2 minutes

Cooking time 0 minutes

Servings: 4

Ingredients:

Lemon slices for garnish, if desired

1 medium sprig of fresh rosemary

Ice cubes

1/6 cup of honey

1/2 large sprig of fresh rosemary for garnish, if desired

2 large strips of lemon peel

1 tbsp of fresh ginger root, grated

Juice of 2 lemons

Directions

Combine sprigs of fresh rosemary, lemon peel, ginger, and honey and add 1 cup of water to a small pot.

Stirring regularly, bring the mixture to a boil, then simmer for about 10 minutes over low heat.

Cool for about 15 minutes, then strain the mixture into a large pitcher. Discard the rosemary and ginger.

Mix together the 2 cups of lemon juice and 3 cups of cold water in a pitcher.

To serve, pour over ice with a lemon slice and a little piece of fresh rosemary as a garnish, if desired.

Nutrition: Calories 69, fat 6.5 g, fiber 2.6 g, carbs 10.6 g, protein 9.4 g Cholesterol: 0mg

Conclusion

Congratulations on making it to the end!

Almost all of us will experience constipation, abdominal pain, bloating, gas, or the inability to pass gas at some point in our lives. The question is, what should we do in such a situation? The quick and easy solution is to take a pain reliever or suck on an antacid. But we don't realize that pain relievers and antacids can only mask the symptoms.

Consider this: If our body is a house, our colon is its sewage. Consider the consequences of a clogged sewer in your home. You don't want this to happen to your body, do you?

Achieving optimal colon health is a journey that involves both the brain and the gastrointestinal system. Home cures emphasizing drinking more water and colon massaging can help the body eliminate waste and absorb nutrients with less effort. The importance of getting enough sleep cannot be overstated; nevertheless, prioritizing improvements to one's dietary habits and exercise routine should come first. Getting enough shut-eye paves the way for eating right and working out regularly. Get a full night's sleep every day, preferably in one stretch. During sleep, our bodies repair and restructure themselves in preparation for the following day. If you think you may be having intestinal problems, a dinner of watery foods may assist.

If you have a colon problem that has been bothering you for a while, you should take it seriously. Learn from the manual's lessons and put them into practice daily.

Keeping your colon healthy is a simple task. It does not necessitate the use of any supplements or laxatives. All you have to do is watch what you eat and get some exercise every day. It shouldn't have been too difficult.

Good luck!

Thank you!

Thank you for making it to this point!

Dear reader,

I am writing to request that you take a few minutes to leave a review after reading my book. I have put a great deal into creating this work, and it is only with the help of thoughtful feedback from readers like yourself that I can continue to refine and improve my writing. So if you have enjoyed my book, I would be truly grateful if you could take a moment to post your thoughts online. Whether you loved it or had a few constructive criticisms, your feedback will help me become a better writer over time. Thank you in advance for your support.

I hope to hear from you soon.